KAREN A. DALEY

OVERCOMING
Stories of Leadership, Resilience, and Action

Overcoming, published November, 2025
Editorial and proofreading services: Cath Lauria; Gina Sartirana
Interior layout and cover design: Howard Johnson
Photo Credits: front cover image by Vecteezy: *vecteezy_ai-generated-minimalist-patterns-background_42191494.jpg*

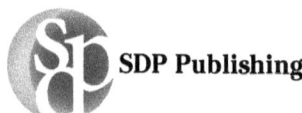 SDP Publishing

Published by SDP Publishing, an Imprint of SDP Publishing Solutions, LLC.

All rights reserved. No part of the material protected by this copyright notice may be reproduced or utilized in any form or by any means, electronic or mechanical, including photocopying, recording, or by any information storage and retrieval system, without written permission from the copyright owner.

Note: The scenarios in this book reflect the author's recollection of events.

To obtain permission(s) to use material from this work, please submit an email request with subject line: SDP Publishing Permissions Department.

Email: info@SDPPublishing.com.

ISBN-13 (print): 979-8-9987414-5-6
ISBN-13 (ebook): 979-8-9987414-6-3

Copyright © 2025, Karen A. Daley

Printed in the United States of America

Dedication

To Eric, whose kindness, care, and friendship have helped me navigate and overcome one of the most challenging periods of my life. To Mary, whose mentorship, wisdom, and guidance have influenced, steadied, and inspired me throughout my life and career.

To Lynn, whose resilience and ability to overcome always astounded me. Rest in peace.

Table of Contents

Foreword 7

Introduction 9

CHAPTER

1 *My Early Home Life* 13
2 *New Beginnings* 19
3 *From Hurt to Finding a Path for Healing* 29
4 *A Career Changing Injury* 35
5 *Injury and Infection Aftermath* 41
6 *A Third Overcoming* 47
7 *Launch of a National Safety Campaign* 53
8 *Forging a New Career Path* 63
9 *ANA Presidency: Part One* 71
10 *ANA Presidency: Part Two* 85
11 *Leadership Lessons Learned* 97
12 *Conclusion* 107

Acknowledgments 113
About the Author 115
References 117

Foreword

Having worked closely with Karen Daley, I was well aware of her story. Yet, I found *Overcoming* so engrossing that I read it in one sitting. Not only did I learn more about Karen's journey, but I was reminded of her commitment, courage, and resilience throughout her career. It's easy to review Karen Daley's many accomplishments through the lens of a PhD-prepared nurse who served as the president of the American Nurses Association. But, as Karen shares, her patient advocacy and leadership in strengthening the profession and healthcare started much earlier.

By sharing her story, Karen reminds us that extraordinary acts of leadership are possible, even in the most challenging of circumstances, if we dare to act. This book is more than a story about Karen's challenges and the impact that she has made. It is a roadmap reminding us all of the power we have in all practice settings, that leadership often emerges in times of adversity if we take action, and that advocacy for ourselves and others is necessary to improve the systems in which we live and work. Few of us will encounter something as devastating as a preventable injury and subsequent life-altering disease that instantaneously alters our career pathway. Karen's choice not to wallow in the situation but rather to advocate for better is both instructional and inspirational. Her commitment to going beyond and applying leadership lessons in advocating for changes in needlestick legislation reminds us that real change often necessitates making structural changes at a societal level.

I vividly remember sitting in my office as Karen and I discussed changes needed to make the American Nurses Association more relevant and responsive to contemporary nursing practice. Karen knew these changes would not be popular or easy, yet her commitment to doing what was right, despite the personal risk of not being reelected for a second term, was evident. That leadership commitment—to do what is right, even when it is difficult—is available to all of us.

Karen is living proof that we have the opportunity to be our best selves even when life throws us an outrageous curveball. Karen's story reminds us that courage and commitment are available for anyone who wants to make a meaningful difference in the world and summons us to serve as advocates and leaders in our own practices and communities.

—**Marla J. Weston**, PhD, RN, FAAN

Introduction

In many ways, the passage of more than fifty years in my career seems like one big blur. Other times, moments appear in my mind as clearly as if they just occurred. Some of those memories and moments throughout my life can still bring emotions to the surface without warning. Reflecting on it all, I am filled with an overwhelming gratitude for opportunities I never could have envisioned for myself.

It is 2025, and healthcare in America is at a critical juncture. At its best, healthcare is about caring for people in a way that is compassionate and responsive to their needs. At its worst, the healthcare system is disorganized, chaotic, and prioritizes the bottom line with inadequate attention paid to the vulnerabilities and needs of those providing and receiving care. Regardless, I cannot imagine caring and effective healthcare without nurses. For more than five decades, I have been one of the millions of registered nurses in this country who have worked to improve people's health. If I had to do it all over again, I wouldn't change a thing despite having suffered a serious and preventable injury on the job that threatened my life. That injury also signaled the end of my time caring directly for patients.

Nursing has been as much a part of who I am at my core as any of my physical characteristics. I loved my years caring for patients, and over time I became an expert nurse and leader. Given my upbringing, I am not surprised I chose nursing as a profession. In many ways, a dysfunctional family history made it a natural fit. I believe many nurses and members of "helping professions" arrive at their career choice as one means to try to fix what they felt powerless to resolve during their childhood. For some like me, it represented a kind of do-over.

The idea of writing this book has existed somewhere in the back of my mind for over two decades, but I have always resisted following through. I have never liked talking about myself—one of the residual effects of my life being raised in a dysfunctional home. Now, as I look back and reflect, I know I have overcome much in my life—not the least of which was a sharps injury I sustained on the job that signaled the end of my nursing career as I knew it at the time. I have never wanted to see myself—or my nursing career—defined solely by that injury. At the same time, I realize my injury story has relevance as a cautionary tale for every practicing nurse and healthcare worker in this country.

I also appreciate the inspirational power and value of sharing personal life stories. The stories I share from my life and career are not intended for you to compare directly with your own, but rather to suggest your own potential to overcome adversity as well as develop as a leader. Opportunities and experiences in leadership may present themselves as job openings in your clinical unit, involvement in staff committees, considerations around returning to school, or connections you intentionally make with other nurses or mentors to help explore your career options.

Over my more than fifty years as a nurse, I have assumed a variety of leadership roles. Beyond singular instances of leadership that I have shared throughout this book, I have also been a leader within my clinical settings and beyond. Some roles I was assigned to; some I volunteered for; some I was elected to; others I applied for and was hired to perform. The culmination of my leadership career occurred with my election in 2010 as president of the American Nurses Association. Today I serve on the board of several healthcare organizations and continue to be invited to speak publicly on topics like sharps injury prevention and leadership.

Leadership is a discussion topic raised by faculty in classrooms across all levels of nursing education and training. For practicing nurses with a desire for career advancement, it is likely an intentional focus. While I do not have specific recall of initiating such discussions or intention during my education, training, and practice, I know from the desire I always had for continuous learning—in whatever form it took—that the wish to grow and excel as a nurse influenced my maturation and career advancement.

If you had the opportunity to speak with nurse leaders around the country about advancement of their careers, they would probably describe taking many different paths. Those paths might include advancing education, progression up clinical ladders, and specialty certifications. They might also describe qualities recognized along the way attributed to good leaders. The ability to demonstrate open listening, empathy, and respect engenders trust among co-workers and allows them to feel heard, seen, supported, and valued by their leaders.

Beyond those qualities, as a leader I have most valued continuous learning, including that gained from academic institutions and educational conferences, being open to new opportunities and responsibilities that allowed me to grow, and the steadying influence and wisdom of mentors.

Born leaders are described as individuals with an innate or natural ability to lead others. People often trust and follow them because they are charismatic, inspirational, nonjudgmental listeners, and passionate about their work. If you think that because you don't identify yourself as a born leader you can't be one, I encourage you to think again. Leaders can also be made or developed by seeking out continuous learning and advancement opportunities, focusing on self-improvement, and learning from experiences and others around them.

We know that nurse leaders can significantly improve the safety and quality of patient care. They enhance its efficiency and effectiveness as they use critical thinking to ensure safe and appropriate actions are taken to improve outcomes for patients. Whether as a member of a team providing direct care or as a leader guiding members of a team, good leaders contribute to productivity and positive practice environments. At the level of organizational leadership, those same skills foster better team engagement as well as healthier processes and outcomes for patients.

Among other things at the intersection of overcoming and leadership—the two main themes of this book—lies resilience. Resilience is about getting back up after you are knocked down. It is the ability to navigate and overcome obstacles and difficult circumstances. It is about maintaining a positive attitude through stressful circumstances and using challenges or negative experiences as an opportunity to become an even stronger person. Resilience is both a skill and an attitude critical for nurses as they do their best to provide care to patients amid healthcare environments that can be chaotic, demanding, and pressure-packed. Estimates I have seen of the percentages of nurses leaving practice within the first two or three years suggest we could be losing a third or more of recent graduates during that period. That level of turnover speaks to the need for employers to help alleviate negative conditions driving nurses out of practice. As I write this book, I find myself thinking that integrating resilience-building skills should be just as much of a priority in today's nursing curricula as building competencies related to critical thinking, problem-solving, and development of practice skills.

Although our personal and professional lives may differ, I believe we have more in common than differences. We all experience struggles and encounter obstacles in our lives. We all must develop the capacity to overcome, to adapt, and to move past them. As I confronted each difficult circumstance in my life, I was faced with choices in how I dealt with it so I could move forward. I am mindful of how overcoming personal adversities throughout my life helped shape the person I became as well as my nursing career and leadership journey.

Writing this book has allowed me to examine and share aspects of my life's circumstances and lessons that have been meaningful for me along the way. I believe this book can serve as an inspirational memoir for those striving to overcome personal and professional challenges.

It has also been written as a leadership memoir with nursing students and practicing nurses in mind. Personal reflections I have shared about my life, career, and leadership experiences are offered with the hope that as you read my story, you will find some inspiration for your own journey.

Chapter

1
▼

My Early Home Life

I have often been asked why I chose nursing as a career. Normally I respond by talking about my mother's illness with diverticulitis that necessitated numerous hospitalizations and surgeries while I was still young. It is true that my consciousness of the work and value of nurses occurred during her hospitalizations. On more than one occasion, I can recall sitting in the hallway watching nurses move between rooms as they tended to patients. For the first time, I wondered about nursing as a possible career—the work seemed so important and meaningful. However, as I reflected further, I realized that memory was only part of that story.

One of my more vivid childhood experiences happened around the time I turned seven. After spending a year in an area hospital recovering from tuberculosis, my father was finally discharged home. During the first few weeks after he returned home, my mother continued to leave in the early morning to work in the coffee shop he owned that was located at the Exchange Building on the Boston Fish Pier. One morning, still early in my father's recovery, he sent me to a nearby store for milk. To reach the store, which was a short distance away, I had to cross a main road that was also a major thoroughfare for traffic in Quincy.

As I was paying for the milk, the elderly woman working the cash register noticed I was alone and said to me, "I don't want you crossing the street on your own. I will take you across."

As she held my hand, a city bus stopped to let us cross. We stepped off the curb and began crossing in the direction of oncoming traffic, which had also stopped. At the same time, the operator of a second city bus drove around the stopped bus into the oncoming lane and hit us both without having time to apply the brakes.

The storekeeper was thrown about twenty feet in the air and sustained serious injuries to her pelvis, hips, and head. I was knocked unconscious with a serious head injury, later diagnosed as a basilar skull fracture that resulted in hearing loss in my right ear for several months. I spent about two weeks in the hospital's pediatric unit being cared for by nurses, one of whom was my cousin Ann. It was her kindness and caring that eased my fears and loneliness, making the time there more bearable and exposing me once more to the difference nurses could make.

I was raised as one of seven children in a two-parent middle-class Irish Catholic family. My youngest sibling—number seven—was my sister Ruth, who was conceived later and no doubt unexpectedly when my mother was forty. Not a lot of family planning was happening in those days with rhythm being the main contraception method recommended by the Catholic church for preventing pregnancy. Based on the number of large families at that time—our neighbors across the street had eleven children—it was not a very effective birth control method. As the fifth child, I was seven or eight years younger than my oldest brother. Although there was only about fifteen years between the oldest and youngest of us, it seemed at times, based on our varied experiences, like we were raised in different families.

By all outward appearances, we looked like a normal family. My parents fed us, clothed us, sent us to school, and provided us with a stable roof over our heads. We lived in a single-family home in a suburb south of Boston on a street with other families who had similar backgrounds and kids who were close to our own ages. Neighborhood kids played with one another, and their parents opened their homes to us. Those who knew me would likely describe me as quiet and serious as a child, but I also loved to laugh and have fun. During the summer months, I would spend much of my time at the municipal park where I could run around, swing, and play softball. During my elementary school years, I often stayed after the last class to help with whatever chores the nuns would find for me to do. Anything but go home.

Regardless of how it appeared from the outside, my early home life was chaotic and largely absent of parental nurturing. My positioning as a middle child often left me feeling a bit invisible—particularly as three of my four brothers began to abuse drugs and alcohol in their early teens. The chaos that ensued was compounded by my parents' alcoholism and their inability to parent in a way that outwardly demonstrated caring emotions. I worked hard, did well in school, and generally stayed out of trouble except for occasional fights with my sister, who was thirteen months older and had special needs. Those fights typically ended with me being punished as the instigator since, as my mother often pointed out, "I should have known better."

From an early age, the primary role I assumed in my family was that of a peacemaker. I can remember, on occasions when my parents would go out, cleaning up the house in an attempt to minimize the alcohol-fueled tensions that would sometimes erupt between my parents after they returned home. Emotions I experienced as a child in my home were dominated by free-floating anxiety and fear. My biggest fear was that one of my parents would get angry and lash out at one of us—not necessarily physically, but emotionally.

It happened unpredictably. Getting the cold shoulder or being yelled at and punished were the most frequent consequences for my misbehavior. Typically, my punishment would result in being banished to an upstairs bedroom for an undefined period. I think I actually enjoyed the peace and quiet in those moments. I learned to spend that time finding creative ways to pass the time, like undressing and redressing the clothes on the Infant of Prague statue that sat on my parents' bureau.

Screaming matches between my parents were not unusual in our home—especially in the evening after drinking. I can recall on many occasions being woken from sleep by one of their fights. I would fearfully sit at the top of the stairs to listen to what was happening to make sure things did not escalate beyond yelling. I am not sure what I thought I could do if things did escalate, though.

One evening, a local parish priest who heard their yelling from the Catholic rectory located a few hundred feet behind our house showed up unannounced. He sat both my parents down to tell them—under the threat of having their kids taken away—that they needed to get sober. He strongly suggested that they start attending Alcoholics Anonymous meetings and pointed out that weekly meetings were held in our parish school hall. That day was the last time my father drank.

It took my mother another year to get sober, and she did so with the help of Alcoholics Anonymous (AA). She remained an active member of AA for more than fifty years and helped many people get sober. I developed a special relationship with that priest, who was later elevated to Bishop of the archdiocese and showed up unannounced at my nursing school graduation. He also carried my high school picture in his wallet for many years.

I believe few people or circumstances could have held as powerful an influence on my parents' drinking as that parish priest did. In many ways, the Catholic Church and their faith were unequaled as potent motivators for my parents. As children, my siblings and I were all enrolled in the Catholic elementary school connected to our parish church which was located behind our home. I also attended a Catholic high school and nursing school. My father, who expected us all to attend weekly confession and Sunday Mass, would quiz us after we came home about which priest said the Mass and what the sermon was about. That worked until we reached our early teens and learned we could just as easily leave Mass early and spend the rest of our Mass time at the Mug and Muffin—a local breakfast place down the street.

Even after both of my parents got sober, however, our home environment remained tense and reactionary, especially as my brothers' alcohol and substance abuse escalated. My father, in particular, could be emotionally volatile and, at times, resorted to physically abusing my brothers as they used alcohol and drugs to self-medicate in the face of a dysfunctional home life. I recall on one occasion yelling at my father to stop beating my brother, who had come home drunk. I still remember my fear as I screamed at him to stop. I thought that he was going to kill my brother and die of a heart attack in the process.

Given my home environment, it would not surprise most to learn that, as a child, I became self-reliant, independent, and overly responsible—inappropriately so at such a young age. In many ways, the personality traits I had developed served me well into my early adulthood. Among other things, I had a keen intuitive sense and empathy that was likely related to constantly walking on eggshells at home and the need to be on alert for the calm to suddenly be breached by angry outbursts or behavior.

I recall sitting at the breakfast table with my siblings, trying not to make any noise so we could leave for school before my mother woke up and came down into the kitchen. Self-protection became paramount for all of us. It emerged as one of the ways I coped and survived an unhealthy upbringing as I left home to attend nursing school.

In many ways, the traits I developed in my childhood represented my first overcoming. In other ways, they stunted my emotional growth as I entered adulthood.

Chapter

2
▼

New Beginnings

I thrived in my nursing program—not always academically, but certainly socially—and in my clinical training. Living in the dorm created another family for me where behavior seemed more predictable and less chaos reigned. I made friends, got involved in extracurricular and other social activities, and, in my senior year, was elected a class officer. I also never missed an opportunity to party.

I frequently left the dorm to go downtown to a club with classmates even in the face of the need to study for a test scheduled for the next day. I have classmates who recall, with mild irritation, my returning from a club to find them studying in the kitchen and sitting down with them to ask, "What did you learn?" Often, my grade on the next day's test would be higher than theirs despite all their studying the night before.

My memories of those times are positive ones punctuated with hard work as well as lots of laughter and fun. Those experiences helped me begin my nursing career less bogged down by my traumatic childhood memories and more confident and excited about the future. In many ways, and for the first time, I felt free to make my own decisions and mistakes without the fear of being unfairly criticized or judged. Diploma program faculty helped guide my development and learning in school. In addition, the wide range of clinical experiences and training I received in school helped prepare me to adapt more quickly in my role as a nurse.

At graduation, I recall my pride in having made it through such a demanding educational program. I also felt happy and excited to begin my career. I had already been hired for my first job as a nurse weeks before graduation. In contrast to the experience of today's new nurse graduates, I went to work at the first and only hospital to which I had applied for a job. After graduation, I moved out of my parents' house and into a home I shared with two friends from school. I also bought my first car—an orange Volkswagen convertible with a white racing stripe along the side. In that driver's seat, I was no longer invisible.

One of my first recollections as a new nurse in 1973 was walking up the ramp to the front entrance into the lobby of the Peter Bent Brigham (PBB) Hospital in Boston (aka the Brigham) with its high ceiling, pillars, and ornate decor. I chose this hospital as my first employer after being exposed to it while watching a movie during one of my classes that described its proud history and showed nurses walking up the ramp wearing their caps, white uniforms, and capes. Established in 1913 as a teaching hospital affiliated with Harvard Medical School, it was renowned for its historic achievements in medicine, most notably performing the first successful kidney transplant from a living donor in 1954.

As I stood mesmerized in that lobby on my first day, I remember telling myself I would work there for two years and then move on to new places and experiences. I did not know at that moment that I would spend my entire twenty-six-year clinical career in this one place. I had no ability at that time to anticipate the many wonderful learning experiences I would have during that time that contributed to my professional identity and growth as a nurse, along with an unexpected workplace event that totally disrupted my career plans.

As a new nurse hire, I was assigned to a women's surgical floor. I began my new job feeling a bit nervous, uncertain of exactly what I would face. It was a challenging environment in which to practice and learn, not only due to the complicated surgeries many of the patients there underwent, but also its unusual physical layout. The thirty-two-bed floor included one private room often used for patients requiring isolation, two semi-private rooms, a nine-bed "small ward" where the most acutely ill surgical patients were cared for, and an open "large ward" with eighteen beds where patient privacy was protected only by curtains.

By today's hospital standards and based on privacy and infection control needs, you would never see anything similar. The best way I can describe it is as a large open room with a sink and countertop area in the middle and eighteen beds positioned next to one another separated by only a bedside table and curtains.

Apart from myself and one other new graduate at that time, the unit nursing staff were more experienced and very supportive. I learned so much in those early months. Relatively soon, my experiences and training allowed me to experience steady growth as a nurse and leader. Within ten months of graduation, I became a day shift charge nurse on the floor—the equivalent of an assistant head nurse—which meant I no longer rotated to evening or night shifts and would assume the role of team leader or be in charge of the entire floor as needed.

As a team leader, I would make patient assignments, pass out meds, and oversee care provided by team members comprised of nurses' aides and other registered nurses. We worked closely with one another as well as with surgical interns, residents, and attending physicians. Part of our routine as a caregiver and charge nurse was to join physician teams on their daily rounds, participating in deliberations as plans were made for patient care and discharge. That culture and work environment promoted confidence in practice and furthered the development of leadership skills in the entire nursing staff, including myself.

Working so closely together with other nurses on that unit provided an opportunity to form many friendships. It was not unusual for some of us to get together for drinks after work. Socializing with others from work who understood the challenges we faced provided a needed outlet. We worked hard, and sharing stories outside of work helped validate our experiences and lessened the pressure we all felt at times. It also brought us closer.

Another place I found the support and growth opportunities I needed was as an active member of my professional organization, the Massachusetts state affiliate of the American Nurses Association (ANA). I had always enjoyed writing, and it was in that space that I first became involved and built self-confidence seeing my articles published in a district newsletter. I was recruited to write articles for another nursing publication that was circulated throughout Boston and later the New England region. I also joined hospital and association committees that were aligned with my personal and professional interests. That was followed by my election to district and state association leadership positions, including serving as president of each.

Each of those experiences brought me together with other nurses, some of whom were leaders and many of whom became lifelong colleagues and friends. They also helped create a network of nurses and mentors who supported me through various phases of my career development and whom I trusted to advise me when faced with situational uncertainty or crossroads in my professional life. Over time, that network made me stronger and more confident as a nurse and nurse leader and allowed me to explore new career directions. It also contributed to my ability to adapt, grow, and become more resilient as a nurse and leader, even after a workplace injury ended my clinical career.

Leadership Story

My first leadership story concerns the care of a frail and petite seventy-year-old woman who had suffered burns over sixty-five percent of her body in a house fire. Based on her age and the extent of her body surface burns, it was more than remarkable that she survived. Her hospitalization included seven months in the ICU and dozens of surgeries. She was transferred to our floor from the ICU where the plan was for her to remain for several weeks. It was there that she would recover from additional surgeries to release scar contractures and skin grafting procedures. Then she would undergo weeks of painstaking physical and occupational therapy before she would finally be ready to go home.

One day, while on walking rounds with the chief of the ward surgical service, he turned to me at her bedside and said, "We will be discharging Bea home in the next couple of weeks." While we had all been expecting it to happen soon, hearing him say it out loud caught me off guard. I was also aware of, based on conversations I had with her, how anxious she felt about leaving the hospital after all this time.

I thought for a minute and responded, "Would you write her a day pass so we can get her out of the hospital today for a few hours?" With physician approval, day passes were occasionally allowed for patients at that time. Those were different days. He agreed without hesitation, understanding that it might help lessen her anxiety a bit about being discharged from the place where she had lived and been so dependent for so many months.

It was the Christmas holiday season, and the surgery schedule, as well as our patient census, was light that week. I enlisted the help of one of our LPNs, wrapped Bea up in a bunch of bath blankets, and sat her in the front passenger seat of my VW convertible. I asked Bea where she wanted to go, and she replied, "I want to see the nativity scene on the Boston Commons." So off we went.

For those unfamiliar with Boston Commons, it is a large city park—over fifty acres of land bordered on each side by major roadways. The nativity scene was positioned in one far corner of the park, but still visible at an angle from the road. I drove around the park several times, but Bea—who was unable to turn her head in any direction due to scarring on her neck—could still not see it.

Not wanting to disappoint her, I did what I needed to do. I drove my car right up over the curb and onto the grass straight toward the nativity scene. Within seconds, I saw blue lights flashing in my rearview mirror and stopped the car. I watched as a Boston police officer got out of his car and walked towards my open driver's side window. As I recall, his first words to me were: "What the hell do you think you're doing?"

I pled my case quickly. "We are nurses from the Peter Bent Brigham taking a patient who has been in the hospital for eight months out for a few hours, and the one thing she wanted to do was see the nativity scene on the Commons." Turning to Bea, I continued: "She couldn't see it from the road because of her burn scars, so I was trying to make it possible for her."

He took a long look at me and then at Bea and said, "Follow me." He got back in his cruiser, turned his blue lights back on, and pulled out in front of us to guide us directly over the grass to the nativity scene. It was the best day ever for all of us, including Bea. She was discharged home about three weeks later.

The initiative I took on Bea's behalf represented an attempt to accomplish a necessary outcome—to lessen her anxiety about her impending hospital discharge. My action was based on my assessment of who she was as a person and her needs at that particular point in time. It can be challenging for nurses as we work to meet the complex range of patients' needs. In this case, I focused on her needs in that moment and the opportunity I saw to respond to it.

While the circumstances and opportunities in this case were pretty unique, nurse leaders use skills, knowledge, and innovative ideas to problem-solve every day as they provide care to their patients. As I think back on my time on that surgical floor, it was there that I made my transition from being a new graduate to becoming a competent and skilled nurse clinician and leader.

Role Transitions

In late 1974, following the announcement that plans were being made to open the first step-down unit at PBB, I applied for my next position—again as a charge nurse on the day shift. The physical design of this unit was so unlike my previous floor, composed of two adjoined wings with all single or semi-private rooms. It was also different with respect to patient acuity and population. Utilized by every in-hospital surgical and medical service, patient admissions most often were ICU, CCU, or Emergency Department transfers with few established criteria guiding utilization.

Patient acuity levels were high and included patients on ventilators and cardiac monitors, some fresh out of acute myocardial infarctions, most with complex medical and post-op needs, and others on investigational drug protocols to manage life-threatening ventricular arrhythmias. The breadth and depth of patient conditions presented a steep learning curve for nursing staff as well as unit leaders like myself. In the absence of any central monitoring capabilities on our unit, cardiac telemetry was only visible to staff in the CCU which was located next to us. That arrangement—unthinkable by today's standards—necessitated frequent nursing rounds each shift to adequately assess patients' needs and conditions.

Leadership Story

One of my lasting memories as a nurse leader on the step-down unit concerned care of a retired judge who suffered from a lethal cardiac arrhythmia syndrome with spontaneous and unpredictable episodes of ventricular tachycardia and ventricular fibrillation (VT/VF). In the pre-ICD era, efforts to prevent and manage such episodes were limited to utilizing investigational drug cocktails and led by two of the preeminent US cardiologists in this field, Drs. Bernard Lown and Thomas Graboys, both of whom were attending physicians at PBB. As specialists in the care of patients with lethal arrhythmias, they managed them on our step-down unit using investigational drug protocols.

While under the care of the Lown team—and despite numerous trials of investigational drug cocktail combinations—the judge suffered repeated VT/VF episodes requiring defibrillation. After one such episode, while he was being cared for in the adjacent CCU and in anticipation of his pending discharge once his rhythm stabilized, I was approached by the judge's wife with a request to be taught CPR. I had come to know her well over many months of caring for her husband.

At the time, Lown service physicians did not subscribe to the belief that providing CPR training to patients' family members was advisable, believing it to be too stressful for them. I agreed to teach her CPR as a clandestine activity—no need for the Lown team to be made aware. I also enlisted the participation of the CCU head nurse in her training. By the time the judge was discharged home, she felt—and demonstrated—complete competence in her CPR skills.

Perhaps two months later, we were informed the judge was being transferred up to our CCU from a local hospital after a successful resuscitation following a VT/VF episode at home. The next day, during Lown team rounds, it was revealed that the judge had experienced a syncopal episode witnessed by his wife and that she had performed CPR until paramedics arrived and defibrillated him. Asked by the Lown team how she had learned CPR, she informed them that she had been taught CPR by Barbara and me prior to the judge's last discharge. From that day on, part of the Lown team's approach for care of lethal arrhythmia patients included CPR training for family members.

As I consider this leadership story and its impact, it reminds me that nurses lead when they act in the way they know to be in the best interest of their patients and their families. Sometimes it takes courage and confidence to be a leader. In this case, I simply responded to an unmet need expressed by the spouse of my patient and, in doing so, allowed her to feel more confident in her role as his primary caregiver.

In 1977, I made the decision to transfer as a staff nurse to the Emergency Department (ED) at PBB. The thought of becoming an emergency nurse appealed to me for numerous reasons. In a Level One Trauma Center, I would be challenged in new ways to continue to learn and grow as a nurse clinician. The care environment I encountered was fast-paced and incredibly demanding, both physically and mentally. It required the ability to learn to deal with high levels of stress and shift care priorities based on a constant shuffling of our census, as well as patients' conditions and needs.

The opportunities for continuous learning and growth in that environment never stopped. It was the perfect place for me to practice—until it no longer was.

Leadership Story

The ED saw a large population of cardiac patients. Many presented with ischemic chest pain, placing them at risk of experiencing or extending a myocardial infarction. For those presenting with ischemic chest pain—which meant the heart muscle was being deprived of oxygen—the standard ED cardiac care protocol included continuous monitoring, sublingual nitroglycerin (nitro), O_2, morphine, beta blockers, and anti-arrhythmics as needed. In the late 1970s, however, what was missing from routine care administered in the ED today for those not responding to other interventions was IV nitro.

Based on established care protocol in the hospital, administration of IV nitro was always accompanied by arterial lines for close monitoring of systolic blood pressure. Since A-line placement was a rare and not routine procedure in the ED, our care protocol for ischemic chest pain stopped short of IV nitro administration. Unfortunately, that meant that patients whose chest pain did not respond to care provided in the ED needed to wait to receive IV nitro until they were admitted into a CCU or ICU bed where an A-line could first be placed. That time delay could also mean the heart muscle was being put at risk of sustaining irreparable damage from a heart attack. I never felt comfortable with that fact.

At that time, evidence validated the accuracy of calibrated automatic BP cuffs which were in common use in our ED. Knowing that, I approached the ED nurse manager with a proposal to work with CCU leadership to create a new protocol that would pilot the use of automated cuffs as the means for closely monitoring blood pressure in patients receiving IV nitro in the ED. She supported the proposal, as did CCU leadership and staff.

The pilot was successful. Next was the addition of IV nitro to our standard ED protocol. That was the place where staff resistance emerged. Still anxious about the safety of administering IV nitro in the absence of A-line monitoring, staff openly expressed ongoing opposition. Regardless, nursing staff followed the new protocol. Within several months, as patient safety was consistently demonstrated, resistance ceased. For me, the experience represented an important lesson in managing and overcoming resistance to change—one that required clear and frequent communication, managing emotions and expectations, involving and empowering staff, and building trust.

Chapter

3
▼

From Hurt to Finding a Path for Healing

By my mid-thirties, while still working in the ED, several issues were becoming apparent to me. In my professional life, I was having a difficult time caring for patients who were drunk or alcoholics. In my dating life, I would experience a feeling of anxiety if I found myself getting too close in a relationship. Demands for more attention or a commitment from the men I was dating felt like smothering and often precipitated a breakup. Thinking back, with one exception, I was the one who initiated those breakups. Finally, I noticed a persistent feeling of resentment and discomfort simmering beneath the surface whenever I spent time around my parents. Regardless of any success in my professional life, my awareness of those feelings created enough discomfort to finally motivate me to seek therapy. As the expression goes, I was sick of being sick and tired.

A Second Overcoming

My brother Kevin, who was about two years older and had moved in with me for several months after he separated from his wife, was already in therapy and struggling with some of the same issues I faced from childhood. We would often stay up into the night talking about our memories, and I shared with him things I was dealing with emotionally. Even as a relatively successful adult, I had begun to realize many of the tendencies and coping skills I developed to survive my childhood no longer served me. In fact, many got in my way. The time had come when I was finally ready to confront my emotional dysfunction.

Kevin recommended his therapist to me, and I began weekly hour-long therapy sessions soon after. Talking about my experiences and feelings as a child was incredibly painful and uncomfortable, like pulling a scab off an old wound. I hated going to therapy sessions because I knew how difficult they were for me to get through emotionally. I often cried in those sessions, which was difficult after living for so long with a protective shell around my feelings. I felt like I was emotionally falling apart. In some ways I was. To begin healing, I needed to reconnect with my true feelings.

Therapy helped me identify the negative messages I had internalized from my childhood. Many drove aspects of my outward personality and behaviors. While I was becoming confident as a nurse, in private I felt a lot of emotional turmoil. As a child, I never felt deserving of love, as my emotional needs were readily dismissed. I carried with me and shared explicit childhood memories that reinforced that message. I also learned at an early age not to cry regardless of what might have precipitated it. Even crying after a physical injury, my parents would often respond by saying, "Stop crying or I will give you something to cry about."

While still in elementary school, one Saturday I recall falling off my bike, getting all scraped up, and knocking out a front tooth in the process—root and all. My friend's mother wrapped the tooth in a wet paper towel and, instead of taking me home, I begged her to take me directly to a dentist. I remember wanting to have my tooth fixed without telling my parents what had happened. I feared being yelled at and punished.

I had learned pretty early as a child that it was better to be invisible and out of the crosshairs of my parents' anger. I became independent and an overachiever. I kept my feelings and personal life private.

I can't remember once bringing a friend home from school. I learned to find positive attention and caring in other places—at school, from parents of my neighborhood friends, and from other adults outside my immediate family. I think my parents were somewhat aware of that need, as they often arranged for me to stay with my grandmother or my favorite aunt and uncle for days at a time. And if awards were given for people pleasing, I would have earned many. Regardless and often to no avail, I still made attempts to please my parents.

It wasn't long into my therapy sessions that the therapist suggested I begin attending Al-Anon meetings. Different than Alcoholics Anonymous, Al-Anon is a self-help group for those who are being impacted by the problem drinking of others. Even though my parents no longer drank, I needed help to overcome the many ways I had been emotionally affected. In those meetings, for the first time, I heard others share experiences and feelings like mine, along with ways to cope.

Early on, I also attended Al-Anon speaker conferences to help me gain better insight into the ways my parents' alcoholism had affected me. I recall in one of those conferences, hearing a particular speaker say to the audience, "What happened wasn't your fault." It was like she was speaking directly to me. Those words opened up something in me, and I found myself sitting there crying uncontrollably. I still carried the burden of responsibility for the dysfunction happening in my childhood home, and I was hurting myself in the process.

I attended meetings on a regular basis for close to a decade. It was in those meetings that I learned new tools for coping and new ways to live regardless of the behaviors of others around me. More than anything, I began to understand that I no longer needed to look beyond myself for what I could control or change. I learned that it was not others' behaviors or illnesses that were the problem, but rather my reaction to them.

The spiritual nature of healing I gained in Al-Anon came not from religion, but from my acknowledgment that I was no longer in charge or needed to try to control people or situations that were not mine to control. All I could control was myself—my own attitudes, reactions, and behaviors. I no longer needed to protect myself. In fact, allowing myself to open up and be vulnerable also allowed me to develop closer personal relationships. Therapy and Al-Anon meetings helped me realize those things, and for the first time in my life, I could begin to live my life in a healthier, happier way.

A necessary part of my healing process, it took me years to realize and accept that my parents did their best given their circumstances growing up. Both of my parents had suffered terribly in their childhoods. While my father never spoke about it, he had been abused both emotionally and physically by his father, an angry and abusive alcoholic who never got sober. My mother was raised in an emotionally repressive home and struggled her entire life to gain some sense of approval or caring from her mother. Both of my parents turned to alcohol to cope. Their drinking was one of the few things they had in common when they married. Years later, I can recall sitting alone one day in the kitchen with my mother when out of the blue she shared with me that she and my father should never have married.

Hearing such a personal revelation from my mother was unusual. I recall feeling shaken as I thought about its meaning. None of my siblings or I would have been born had my parents never been married. It also likely reflected some of my mother's emotional regret for the years we all suffered as the result of their oft-times toxic relationship and marriage.

In his eighties, my father was diagnosed with pancreatic cancer. By the time surgery was performed at an area city hospital, his tumor was too advanced to remove. The surgeon simply closed him back up. He called me at home the next morning to tell me my father did not want any further treatment. Per his wishes, pain management would become their main priority. Knowing his time was short, I contacted all my siblings—many of whom lived out of state—to suggest they travel home if they wanted to see him and say goodbye. One by one, they did.

A few days after his surgery, I was sitting by his bed in his hospital room while he lay there awake, but staring off into space. I asked him, "Dad, what are you thinking about?"

Very uncharacteristically, he said, "I'm thinking about all the things I would do differently if I had the chance." I didn't probe any further, but I knew at that moment he was apologizing to us all. It also occurred to me at that moment that he knew he was close to death and might find comfort in spending his final days in a Catholic hospital in the Boston area.

I asked the hospital staff to make the necessary arrangements, and he was transferred there the following day. The hospital accommodated my request for a private room to allow all of us to freely visit and sit with him around the clock. While the morphine drip provided him with needed pain relief, it was also causing him to hallucinate and become confused.

To avoid any need for staff to physically restrain him, I stayed with him the last few nights. Whenever he got agitated or started trying to get out of bed, hearing my voice and feeling my hand on his arm would be enough for him to relax and lie back down. Being able to do that for him brought me needed comfort in the face of my own grief. He died peacefully a couple of days later, about two weeks after he had been diagnosed with cancer.

My mother, ten years younger than my father, experienced a longer period of health decline. In her late seventies, it was apparent she was having significant memory issues. My father had passed years before, and she was living alone in an apartment development for seniors. After several episodes of confusion in the middle of the night associated with wandering, not eating, and being found confused behind the wheel of her car, she was finally placed in a nursing home. Over time, her mental status deteriorated to the point of not being able to recognize anyone.

As cruel as dementia can be, in some respects it became a blessing as her protective emotional walls were stripped away. She seemed happy to see us whenever we visited—far cry from the angry, emotional states we encountered in her early days there. One day, during one of my visits, she asked me, "Do you ever see that girl Karen?"

I said, "Yes, I see her a lot."

Her response to me was totally out of character. "She's very nice." It was the first time I could remember my mother speaking to me in a caring way. That moment provided some needed healing for me, and whenever I think of her, it is one of the memories I hold most closely.

My mother lived with dementia for a number of years. As time passed, her physical body failed, and she was placed in hospice care.

During her remaining time, the nursing home and hospice staff treated her with kindness, caring, and dignity.

I was at home one weekend getting ready to drive to the nursing home to visit her when my phone rang. On the phone was a nurse practitioner who told me my mother had just passed. Feeling awful that I was not there when she died, in the next breath she informed me my mother was not alone when she passed and that she had stayed with her. I will always feel grateful for her kindness.

Leadership Reflections

My recognition of the need to change my behaviors and attitudes did not come easily. When those personal realizations did surface, they emerged from my need for some relief from the emotional turmoil I felt. I now know how important it was for my health and well-being that I find a path that would allow me to begin to heal my childhood wounds. I believe that many people struggle against emotional baggage of one kind or another. No life is perfect. The most important thing, once you recognize it, is to take positive steps to heal your pain.

I also recognize that, like many people, I am a work in progress. Engaging in these processes to overcome my hurts and heal my wounds has made me a better person and nurse leader. It has also given me personal insights and a self-awareness that I didn't have before. As part of letting go of negative internal messaging, I can acknowledge that I deserve love and happiness and be more open in my life to receiving care and asking for help from others. None of those was a given prior to beginning this healing process.

Chapter

4

▼

A Career Changing Injury

By the summer of 1998, I had been an ED nurse for more than twenty years. As a senior member of the nursing staff, I remained in a direct care provider role—always my strongest preference and where I felt I made the most difference. I would also be assigned the role of charge nurse for my shifts as needed, working closely with the ED attending physician.

On the day of my injury, I was assigned to triage. It was a typically busy weekend day with a full waiting room and a steady influx of walk-in and ambulance transport patients.

Sharps Injury

About halfway into my twelve-hour shift, one of my nurse colleagues working inside the ED approached me to ask if I could attempt a blood draw on one of her patients. She had already made two unsuccessful attempts and did not want to stick him again. I arranged triage coverage and went to see her patient, an elderly man who seemed confused and dehydrated.

I was able to retrieve the blood samples on the first draw, and as I held pressure on the venipuncture site, I reached behind me to place the contaminated needle into the sharps disposal box on the wall. As I placed the needle into the box positioned above my eye level, a second needle protruding from the overfilled box and out of my view stuck my index finger.

I knew right away from the pain, as well as the blood visible on the outside of my glove, that I had sustained a deep puncture. I have often been asked since my injury how I felt at the moment my injury occurred. My initial reactions ranged from shock to anger to frustration based on the fact that overfilled needle boxes were not uncommon on our unit and had generated a lot of staff complaints. I also wanted to ignore the exposure and just go back to work. The ED was busy, and I did not want to take the time to be seen for a stick that I assessed as low risk, based largely on an air-exposed needle.

Given the nature and depth of my exposure from an unknown source, recommended follow-up would require me to come in on my days off for post-exposure testing, which would create more anxiety as I waited for my results. Additionally, up to six weeks of HIV post-exposure prophylaxis (PEP) might be recommended. Having cared for other nurses prescribed PEP for their exposures, I knew how toxic those drugs could be to healthy individuals. I simply wanted to return to triage, finish the rest of my shift, and pretend it had never happened.

I had been stuck before, perhaps as many as four or five other times over the course of my career. Most of those exposures had occurred in the ED, and I probably had only reported half of them based on my personal assessment of the level of exposure risk. I had previously contracted sub-clinical hepatitis B (HBV), likely related to caring for an infected trauma patient before standard precautions were being routinely observed. That bloodborne pathogen exposure left me with protective antibodies, so HBV was not a concern. But this was 1998—the era of HIV and a new classification of hepatitis initially called non-A, non-B that was now renamed hepatitis C (HCV).

At the same time I was considering ignoring my exposure, the nurse who requested the blood draw and witnessed the needlestick occur said, "I know you are going to sign in and be seen for that. Right?" I always think of her with gratitude as I speak about my injury. I am not sure I would have sought care had she not been there to encourage me to do so.

I signed in and was seen by one of our nurse practitioners (NP). She took my exposure history, examined my puncture site, and following our post-exposure protocol, recommended baseline labs and post-exposure prophylaxis (PEP).

Baseline labs would establish that I was negative for HIV and HCV at the time of my needlestick. PEP was recommended based mainly on the fact that no source patient could be identified. No prophylactic therapy was available at the time for HCV. I deferred taking PEP. It is a decision I regret to this day. There is a high likelihood, if I had taken and tolerated a full course of PEP, I would not have contracted HIV.

So I went back to work and my life as if nothing had ever happened. No mention was made of my exposure by other ED nurses who were aware that it had happened, and that was how I liked it. I worked hard to put my injury out of my mind. I was largely successful in that effort—in fact, too successful—as I resumed work and continued to draw blood, place IVs, and assist with ED procedures involving sharps.

Health Issues

Then things began to change. Within a matter of weeks, I started experiencing vague symptoms. I began to notice unexplained weight loss, fatigue, some loss of appetite, and mild abdominal pain that would come and go. I would leave the ED for my lunch break, and by the time I got to the cafeteria, I'd feel too nauseated to eat. Puzzled, but not seriously alarmed, I initially related my symptoms to the first anniversary of the sudden death of my brother Kevin who had died in a single car crash in July of 1997. I still felt a profound sadness after his loss.

Until that time, my health had consistently been good. By the time I finally saw my primary, I weighed about eight pounds less than I had at my previous annual check-up. I described my symptoms, but didn't mention my sharps injury (SI) from a few months ago. The truth is it never occurred to me that my injury could have had anything to do with the symptoms I was now experiencing. I had put my exposure in the back of my mind soon after it happened.

After taking a history and doing an exam, she said, "Karen, I can see that you've lost weight and that you aren't feeling well. I am going to send off some labs, and if nothing shows up and you continue to feel unwell, you should come back and see me again." Of course, the labs she ordered came back normal.

In the weeks that followed, I continued feeling fatigued and unwell. I never missed a work shift during this period, though. At the time, in addition to continuing to work in the ED, I was also serving as president of the state affiliate of the ANA which was beginning to experience some internal dissension from our labor members. By the time I finally scheduled a second appointment with my primary, about five months after my exposure, I had lost about twelve pounds in combination with my other symptoms. On my way to my appointment that day, and in an attempt to save myself another visit on a day off, I stopped by the Occupational Health Clinic to request to have my six-month follow-up labs be drawn early. As my labs were drawn, I made no mention of the fact that I was on my way to see my primary physician for the second time in a matter of months.

Diagnoses

The following week, I came into work to cover the shift of a co-worker who had to leave unexpectedly due to a family emergency. Once again assigned to triage, it occurred to me in the afternoon that I had not heard back from the Occupational Health (OH) Clinic about my lab results. I called the clinic and they suggested I come by as soon as possible, as the clinic would soon be closing, but that one of the NPs would wait for me. By the time I was able to get there, the clinic was closed, but the door was unlocked. I went in and sat in one of the clinic chairs.

While waiting, I was able to hear someone speaking on the phone behind a closed door. A few minutes later, an NP I had never met before came out of the office, introduced herself, and asked me to come in. She then informed me that my lab tests needed to be redrawn. My first thought was to ask: "Why? Were the samples lost?"

She looked at me, shaking her head, and responded, "No. The tests weren't negative."

Knowing follow-up labs included testing for HIV and HCV, and at a loss for what to say next, I asked her: "Both?"

She responded "yes" and informed me that the repeat labs would be sent to California for more sensitive confirmatory testing. She also told me that rather than have me wait for a call to let me know the results were back, she would schedule a follow-up appointment for me now, at which time I would come back to the clinic to receive the results.

It was about a week later, on Wednesday, December 23, when I returned to the clinic. I can remember walking up from the parking lot, anxious about learning the results and concerned I might run into someone I knew on my way to the clinic.

Not long after I arrived for my appointment, I was called into one of the clinic exam rooms. As I entered the room, the first person I saw was the OH medical director, followed by the nursing director, an NP, a social worker, and an infectious disease (ID) fellow. Walking into that room, it wasn't necessary for them to tell me that my results had been confirmed as positive. For the most part, I am not even sure what was said after that point as I stood there in shock. I do recall, however, something so important that the NP asked me. I heard her say, "What do you need from us?"

Not sure for a moment how to respond, I did make two requests. First, I asked that my name be kept confidential—even from administration. I knew hospital officials would need to be made aware that an employee had been infected after an occupational exposure. They did not, however, need to be told my identity. I had worked at the hospital for a long time and knew I would need time to deal with the news I had just been given. I did not want to be focused on by reassuring friends or colleagues who might reach out after hearing the news. I also did not know at that time the degree to which co-infection with HIV and HCV might pose a serious threat to my health or life.

Second, I asked the ID Fellow if she could refer me to a new primary, an ID specialist outside of the Brigham. At that time, the HIV clinic was the only place where HIV-positive patients were seen at PBB. That would make confidentiality difficult to maintain. Without any hesitation, both requests were honored.

Chapter 5

Injury and Infection Aftermath

Experiencing Uncertainty and Loss

I left the OH clinic in a fog—more like shock, I think. I felt overwhelmed and not sure what to do next to navigate this horrific situation. I had enjoyed good health for most of my life. I was pretty active, had quit smoking long ago, only drank socially, and until recently, had maintained a reasonable weight for most of my life. Perhaps the worst part of my lifestyle was how I ate—not the healthiest from a nutritional standpoint. Now, at the age of forty-six, I was not sure what I faced or whether I would survive it. And despite the fact that progress was being made in HIV care, less was known at that time about HCV. I was also aware that people sometimes died from co-infection with these two viruses.

As I stood at the elevator that would allow me to exit the hospital on the first floor, it suddenly dawned on me that I would never return to the ED. That was not because having HIV precluded it, but because I knew I would be facing rigorous drug therapies and did not think it advisable that I go back to such a demanding setting or work with sharps again. The decision I made following my diagnoses to leave direct care crushed me. I loved working in the ED and considered myself an expert ED nurse.

Just as difficult for me to think about was the fact that I would no longer work alongside many of the ED nurses, who were like family to me. I could not imagine leaving the work or the people I had known, cared about, and socialized with for so many years. That loss lingers despite the passage of time. Not surprisingly, my dreams still take me back there sometimes, and there is always someone in the dream who walks up to me and says, "Karen, you are not supposed to be here."

I drove home knowing I needed to get away. I decided to visit my sister Ruth and her family in North Carolina. She and I were very close despite a seven-year age difference. I called her to let her know I would be visiting on short notice for the Christmas holidays. She didn't ask me any questions about the reason for my sudden visit, but I felt the need to offer some explanation, saying, "They have too many nurses scheduled over the holidays in the ED, so I decided to take time off."

Ruth simply told me she looked forward to seeing me. I hung up and reserved a one-way flight to NC for the next morning. Before I left, however, I knew I needed to let someone I trusted in the ED know what had happened and where I could be reached in case anyone needed to get in touch with me. I called Michael Robinson—a longtime friend and nurse co-worker in the ED whom I totally trusted. I was confident he would keep everything I shared to himself. I also spoke with the ID fellow who would be arranging an outside physician referral while I was away.

I arrived in NC the next day. After a short time, my sister suggested we go out for a drive. Not five minutes later, she pulled the car over and said, "I know they don't have too many staff on during the holidays. What's really going on?"

Not sure how to say it, I just told her outright that I had been infected with HIV and HCV from a needlestick in the ED. I could see the shock and concern on her face. I never got used to seeing that reaction from people.

One afternoon, a couple of weeks later, the phone rang. Ruth answered it and handed it to me, saying, "It's for you." I took the phone, figuring it was either Michael or the Brigham ID fellow.

I was surprised to hear an unfamiliar voice on the other end say, "Hi Karen. My name is Dr. Eric Rosenberg. I am an infectious disease attending physician from Mass General Hospital (MGH), and I will be your new primary care physician. I am just calling you to let you know that you are going to be okay."

Even all these years later, thinking about that moment makes me feel so emotional and grateful. His kind reassurance was just what I needed to hear at that time. I felt my body start to relax for the first time in weeks.

Treatment Begins

I made arrangements to return home soon after so that I could begin my care at MGH. At my first appointment with Eric, we sat in an office for over an hour discussing my care. He took his time with me explaining what he anticipated would be my disease trajectory and his initial approach to treating my co-infection. He had already been in touch with an HCV specialist at MGH with whom I met that same day. Based on my immune function, Eric explained that he believed I would fall into the category of "slow HIV progressor" and mapped out my disease trajectory on a piece of paper. If his prognosis was correct, with good viral suppression, my lifespan could be expected to be close to normal.

Towards the end of our time together, as we were discussing my injury and the HIV drugs he would be prescribing, he wrote something else on a piece of paper and pushed it across the table towards me. Unsure of what I was looking at—the paper contained a series of numbers—Eric said, "That's my home phone number. If you ever find yourself lying awake at three in the morning thinking about this, don't lie there worrying. Call me instead." Knowing I had his number, I never needed to make that call. To this day, Eric remains my infectious disease specialist and treasured friend.

Care for HCV in combination with HIV complicated my disease management. With high amounts of each virus in my blood, the decision was made to treat both viral infections simultaneously. At the time, the only drug regimen for HCV involved daily injections with interferon and ribavirin, an oral antiviral medication. Both carried a significant side effect profile, and the plan, depending on my tolerance, was to keep me on both HCV drugs for an entire year. The HIV drugs would be a lifelong therapy.

The prescribed treatment regimens were difficult—especially in the first few months. I experienced a wide range of side effects, not the least of which were skin rashes, extreme fatigue, anorexia, weight loss, hair loss, lactic acidosis, and chemical hepatitis. A number of them necessitated changes being made to my prescribed HIV therapies.

During that time, I made almost weekly visits to MGH to see Eric and have labs checked due to the difficulty stabilizing my care and tolerance of my HIV treatment regimen. My response to the year-long HCV therapy was also monitored by an MGH hepatologist. That therapy had to be stopped two months short of the intended twelve months due to significant T-cell suppression. Fortunately, those ten months of treatment with interferon and ribavirin were sufficient to permanently eradicate HCV from my system.

Psychological Impact

Aside from the physical side effects of both therapies, I experienced significant psychological stressors in the months after my diagnoses. As the direct result of my infections, I was facing unsettling feelings similar to those I experienced earlier in my life.

As a child, my life was punctuated not only with chaos, but with a frequent sense of unpredictability. Now, as an adult, I found myself once again facing some of those same feelings. Some related to the anxiety and fear I experienced as I waited for my test results, along with an inability to know how my health would be impacted each time my medication regimen needed to be adjusted or changed. One recurring fear I had, particularly in the face of the extreme fatigue and leg weakness I was experiencing from the HCV drugs, related to my worry that I might fall, hit my head, open a bleeding wound, and not be alert enough to warn someone about the bloodborne viruses I carried.

On occasion, I've been asked why I wasn't angrier at my employer—or even God—about what had happened to me. The truth is, I did feel angry at times. Those feelings, however, were short-lived and displaced by other things. I was preoccupied with the physical effects of my treatment regimens and, at the same time, couldn't help but feel grateful that I was being cared for by two of the finest infectious disease and HCV specialists in the Boston area. I've learned that it's hard to feel grateful and angry at the same time.

It also didn't take me long to realize that my occupational injury could have happened anywhere. My employment setting was no different than hundreds of others across the country in that respect. So rather than rail against my employer, I channeled my anger where I felt it could do the most good. I went public with my injury and its horrific consequences and began to travel around the country to raise awareness among healthcare workers, hospital executives, and policymakers about the need for better worker protections. My intention, wherever and to whomever I spoke, was to put a face to the issue of preventable SI and share my own story as a cautionary tale.

The losses I was experiencing burdened me for months and even years after leaving clinical practice. There were times when my losses dominated my thoughts and feelings. Before my injury, my professional life provided me with purpose and meaning. I had caring and valued relationships with friends from my workplace. The disruptions to my health and my clinical career felt overwhelming. I had never before experienced a serious illness. The physical and emotional upheaval I felt at times was unsettling and left me feeling socially isolated and alone. I missed my work and friends at the Brigham. And while I had the support of other friends and family, it was difficult for them to understand what I was going through.

Two things helped me navigate those early months. First, I began journaling again. Journaling was a tool I had begun using while I was in therapy and Al-Anon. It was invaluable in helping me get out and process my feelings. I also read a book recommended to me titled *Working on a Miracle* (Johnson and Olshan 1997). Written by Dr. Mahlon Johnson, a Vanderbilt pathologist, the book chronicles his experience in 1992 after his scalpel slipped while he was performing an autopsy on a patient who had died of AIDS.

During an era when AIDS was still incurable and almost always terminal, his book describes his journey after testing positive for HIV and his persevering efforts to push beyond conventional wisdom and find a cure as he tested new HIV drug combinations on himself. As remarkable and groundbreaking as his scientific contributions were, it was the emotional journey he endured throughout that resonated most strongly with me. For the first time since my injury, another healthcare provider's personal recounting of what he experienced psychologically reassured me that all the emotions I was feeling as a result of my injury and infections were normal. That was a huge gift.

It was perhaps the sense that I had lost who I was as a person that posed the most difficult challenge for me. I even found myself questioning whether I was still a nurse. Caring for patients had made me the person I was, and without that, I felt lost and without purpose. To a large extent, I wasn't sure of my professional identity anymore.

I was reminded of an expression I had heard at an Al-Anon meeting: *When you are what you do, when you don't, you aren't.* So much of my identity and life had revolved around being a nurse at the Brigham, including many of my close relationships. It felt as if my infection with HIV and HCV overshadowed anything else I knew about myself. My illness had now become my identity.

I had received lots of validation throughout my clinical career from co-workers, physicians, and others for being perceived as a good nurse. After I went public with my illness, one of my writing mentors and friends, Judith Mitiguy, authored an article about me that was published in the *Journal of Emergency Nursing*. In it, she referred to me as a *nurse's nurse*. Having that phrase attributed to me by a nurse I respected so much meant a lot. In fact, it meant more than any award or recognition I'd received throughout my career.

Now, instead of feeling centered in the work and profession I loved, my life became consumed with tests, medications, doctor appointments, and not knowing what might come next. I did not want my infections to define my identity, but there was rarely a day—especially in the early months after my diagnoses—when my first thought as I woke in the morning wasn't that I had HIV and HCV.

Chapter 6

A Third Overcoming

The Personal Becomes Public

After the initial shock of learning I was infected with two potentially life-threatening viruses, I largely kept the news to myself. I soon learned how emotionally taxing it was for me to share the information with others. I also knew I needed to conserve my emotional and physical energy to allow me to deal with what was ahead. Side effects of the prescribed therapies were grueling, including bone-numbing fatigue and leg heaviness that made me feel weak on my feet.

For the first few weeks, I had only confided in my closest friends and family. One exception to that was informing a small number of staff leaders at the Massachusetts Nurses Association (MNA) where I continued to serve as president. A few months into my treatment, my labs and health finally began to stabilize. As that happened, I began to think more about the circumstances surrounding my SI, including how it could have been prevented. I began exploring the existing literature and research on SIs—their frequency among healthcare workers, the nature of those injuries, and whether any safer sharps technology was available that might help reduce injuries. What I learned was startling.

Sharps Injuries in 1999

At the time my injury occurred, the Centers for Disease Control (CDC) estimated that healthcare workers sustained approximately 600,000 to 800,000 SIs annually in the US (NIOSH 1999). To my astonishment and alarm, I also learned that safety-engineered sharps devices had existed for decades, but fewer than fifteen percent of hospital employers were providing workers access to even one type of sharps safety device to help prevent injuries.

Evidence also existed to indicate that use of these devices could prevent more than sixty percent of SIs (National Surveillance System for Healthcare Workers 2011). It did not make any sense to me—particularly in this era of potentially life-threatening bloodborne pathogens—that employers were not making them available to their workers.

The first generation of sharps safety devices had been introduced to the market in the late 1980s in response to the HIV epidemic. By the time my injury occurred in 1998, a third generation of safety devices was available, typically designed with sheaths or sliding barrels that required manual activation to cover a contaminated needle before disposal. I also learned that semi-automatic retractable needles had been introduced to the market, but they were in an early phase of development and adoption. I knew that my injury could easily have been prevented by some type of protective needle design, along with better placement of and attention to emptying the overfilled disposal box.

As the federal agency established to help ensure healthy workplaces for American workers, efforts directed by the Occupational Safety and Health Administration (OSHA) to reduce SIs at that time were largely in the form of the Bloodborne Pathogens Standard (BPS). Given the number of US hospitals, on-site inspections were rarely conducted. However, despite the existence of OSHA recommendations for employers to provide access to existing sharps safety technology, few if any incentives existed for them to do so. And in the absence of meaningful OSHA enforcement, most employers ignored that section of the BPS.

Advocacy Begins

Having educated myself about the preventable nature of many SIs, including mine, I approached the MNA Executive Director and the Director of Government and Legislative Affairs (GOVA) to request a bill be filed in the state legislature to promote SI prevention. Prior to that, no such bill had ever been filed in Massachusetts. Around the time of my injury, attention was also starting to be paid by the media to a growing number of healthcare workers being infected on the job with bloodborne pathogens like HIV and HCV.

Of particular note was a three-part series published in 1998 in the *San Francisco Chronicle* on healthcare workers and patients contracting occupational infections due to contaminated sharps against the backdrop of the availability of safety sharps and an ongoing AIDS epidemic. At the time, the CDC mandated all hospital employers to report the occurrence of worker infections due to occupational bloodborne pathogens exposures. Most resulted from SIs. My injury and the resulting infections had been confidentially reported to the Bureau of Infectious Disease and Laboratory Sciences within the Massachusetts Department of Public Health (MDPH).

One day, while at the MNA headquarters in the spring of 1999, I was approached by the GOVA director. The state bill we filed earlier, HB 969, had been assigned to the Joint Health Care Committee and a legislative hearing would soon be scheduled. She informed me that I had a decision to make—whether or not I would publicly testify before the committee in support of the bill.

This decision went beyond simply offering public testimony at the State House. If I made the decision to testify, the plan would be to bring as much public attention as possible to the issue of preventable SIs. To that end, MNA would be sending out a press release in advance of the hearing. That meant I would need to tell others among my family and friends about what had happened to me ahead of any news being publicly released. As nervous as I felt and knowing it was the right thing to do, I agreed to testify.

My family was my first priority. I reached out to my brothers and my older sister, Lynn, who lived with schizophrenia. I had no idea how they would respond to the news, but all were incredibly supportive.

Still, those calls were hard. Next, I thought about informing close friends and co-workers at the Brigham ED. Before meeting with ED staff, however, I scheduled a face-to-face with the Chief Nursing and Medical Officers at the hospital, both of whom I knew personally. Until our meeting, neither had realized that I was the employee who had been infected.

I sat across a conference table from them, explaining how my injury could have been prevented and how it was impacting my health and career. To their credit, they asked me what they could do. Based on our conversation, a needlestick prevention committee was established, and an inventory of hospital sharps was immediately initiated with an eye towards piloting and promoting widespread adoption of safety-engineered sharps devices. Sharps disposal boxes were also repositioned on walls throughout the hospital at an average eye level with additional emphasis placed on the need for staff and management to ensure they were being emptied on a regular basis.

Next, I arranged a face-to-face meeting with the entire ED staff. Many had been wondering why I had been out of work for such a long period. Given the news they were about to hear, I thought it important that I be there in person to reassure them and leave no room for speculation around the state of my health.

It was a very emotional day. I met with everyone in an ED conference room. That included physicians, nurse co-workers, unit secretaries, and other members of the care team, most of whom I had not seen for many months. A few weeks later, the staff presented me with a beautiful bracelet that I continue to wear and treasure to this day. I also wrote a letter explaining my circumstances to the MNA staff that I asked the MNA Executive Director to read on my behalf.

The other action I took in advance of the hearing date was to contact the current ANA president, Dr. Beverly Malone. As a state association president, I would soon be expected to attend a national meeting of state presidents and executive directors hosted annually by ANA in DC. I knew once the legislative hearing took place, word of my injury and health consequences would spread quickly.

I also knew I looked sick at this point—particularly from the hepatitis C drugs. I had continued to lose weight, was still experiencing awful fatigue, my hair was thinning and falling out, and my face had taken on an unhealthy, grayish tint. In my conversation with Dr. Malone, I requested an opportunity to address the Constituent Assembly. She was incredibly kind and supportive and readily agreed.

The Massachusetts Bill

Back in Massachusetts, the day of the legislative hearing on the SI prevention bill we filed finally arrived. As the committee chair announced that they were ready to hear testimony for our bill, I stepped forward to take a seat at the table from which I provided my statement. Later that afternoon, following additional testimony from other representatives of the healthcare community, the bill was reported out favorably by a unanimous vote of the committee.

Despite the fact that I knew we had sent out a press release in advance, nothing prepared me for what I encountered that day—an overflowing hearing room as well as newspaper reporters crowding the outside hallway requesting interviews after the hearing.

Local and Boston media reported on the issue and my story that evening and in the days that followed. One result of that attention from statewide print and television media was the immediate formation of a Needlestick Prevention Advisory Committee by Dr. Howard Koh, the Commissioner of Public Health in Massachusetts. The committee was charged with examining regulatory approaches for reducing needlestick injuries across the state. Dr. Koh appointed me to that committee, and I remain connected to its work to this day.

On August 17, 2000, within one legislative session, An Act Relative to Needlestick Injury Prevention was signed into law in Massachusetts. The new law required the use of safety devices in all Massachusetts hospitals licensed by the Department of Public Health. Compliance with the provisions contained in the new state law was tied to hospital licensure, creating an especially strong incentive for employers to comply. With the passage of this legislation, Massachusetts became the first and only state covered by federal OSHA with mandated hospital reporting of SI data.

Another crucial aspect of the law was creating the first statewide SI surveillance system in the US, collecting data on the nature, method, timing, and location of reported injuries. Since its inception in 2002, all Massachusetts hospitals licensed by MDPH have reported data—an amazing commitment to that safety surveillance system. In the years since 2002, annual summary data reports have been shared with all Massachusetts hospitals, providing an opportunity for employers to improve their own SI prevention efforts.

Chapter

7

▼

Launch of a National Safety Campaign

By the spring of 1999, there were indications that growing attention was being focused across the country on preventable SIs to healthcare workers. California led the way in July 1998 as the first state to pass a law to mandate the use of sharps safety technology. This was followed by the passage of a study bill in Tennessee in early 1999 that directed a review of available safety sharps. The "Deadly Needles" series published by the *San Francisco Chronicle* (Holding and Carlsen 1998) spotlighted the devastating global effect on health and life of preventable bloodborne pathogens exposures, some resulting from the re-use of contaminated conventional needles still in use decades after the introduction of safety-engineered sharps devices.

Around that same time, I had the honor to meet and work with a nurse pioneer from Pennsylvania named Lynda Arnold, who after contracting HIV from a work-related SI, courageously went public and forged a path for reform years before my injury and infection became known. Lynda singlehandedly waged a campaign to enlist hospital leaders' voluntary commitment to utilize sharps safety technology. That same spring, OSHA began collecting data from 300 hospitals willing to participate in a study to evaluate the effectiveness of safety technology in SI prevention.

There were few things of more value to me when it came to professional networking and amplification of critical issues impacting nurses and patients than the connections I made as an active MNA member and ANA state affiliate leader. At the ANA CA meeting in the spring of 1999, I nervously stood before all the state presidents and executive directors and explained what had happened to me. As I finished speaking to those state leaders, I made a sincere but spur-of-the-moment offer saying, "I will go anywhere, anytime, and speak to anyone to prevent what has happened to me from happening to anyone else."

That moment became an important catalyst for a whirlwind of activism on local, state, and national levels. It was also the first step in what would soon emerge as a national campaign for SI prevention led by the ANA.

Susan Wilburn, the Director of Occupational Health and Safety at ANA, immediately assumed a lead role as ANA launched a national campaign to raise awareness of serious risks associated with continued use of conventional needles where safety devices existed. In addition, the ANA Government Relations department began fashioning a new SI prevention bill to put before Congress. ANA had been leading on this issue since the early 1980s when it began lobbying Congress to update the BPS through federal statute. Unfortunately, no movement on the bill had occurred for many years, and the approach taken to date by OSHA in the form of the Standard had been largely ineffective in incentivizing employers to improve sharps safety among their healthcare workers.

Activity across the states ramped up quickly. Soon after I extended my offer to travel anywhere and speak to anyone to raise awareness around the importance of SI prevention, I began to receive invitations from ANA state leaders. Over the next two years, I would travel to many states—some more than once—to meet and speak with nurses, hospital administrators, and state legislators. By the end of 1999, twenty-two states had introduced legislation to reduce and prevent injuries, and laws had been enacted in another five.

Additional factors influenced the political environment. ANA helped convene a powerful coalition of stakeholders to educate employers and pressure federal legislators to take action. Among them were leaders of the American Hospital Association (AHA), specialty nursing organizations, healthcare worker unions, and device manufacturers. Media outlets stayed focused on the problem with an appetite for putting a face to the issue. For myself, in addition to traveling to hold meetings with state legislators or offer presentations to hospital staff to raise awareness, print or televised interviews would often be arranged by state association executive directors to maximize the impact of my visit.

HCV was also now recognized as a serious risk for healthcare workers who sustained SIs on the job, and public media outlets were paying attention. As a leading cause for liver transplants across the US (Chitturi and George 2000, 588–91), HCV was being encountered more frequently as a previously undocumented virus in patients who used IV drugs, often existing as a co-infection with HIV.

Lastly, experiences similar to Lynda Arnold's as well as my own were signaling a need for the healthcare industry and legislators to use their power to enhance current workforce safety policies.

Federal Regulatory and Legislative Activity

In May of 1999, with the urging and support of the ANA, HR 1899, the Healthcare Worker Needlestick Prevention Act of 1999, was introduced by cosponsors Representatives Pete Stark (D-CA) and Marge Roukema (R-NJ). The bill, presented at a press conference held at the US Capitol with the National Press Corps present, was designed to update OSHA's 1991 BPS. Speaking in support of HR 1899 were Representative Stark, the vice president of Kaiser Permanente in California, and the president of the Service Employees International Union (SEIU). I offered a statement on behalf of ANA. Six days later, Senators Harry Reid (D-NV) and Barbara Boxer (D-CA) introduced an identical bill in the Senate.

In June 1999, and in conjunction with the launch of ANA's *Safe Needles Save Lives* campaign, a concerted effort was made by ANA to coordinate injury prevention advocacy activities. Over the next twelve months, the ANA facilitated educational activities that provided nurses across the US with training in the evaluation, selection, and implementation of safer sharps devices in the workplace. On two different occasions in September of 1999, at ANA's invitation, I made the trip back to Washington DC.

The first occasion was an educational briefing where I shared my injury experience with the Congressional Women's Caucus. By that time, HR 1899 had secured bipartisan support from 120 House sponsors and from a coalition of more than thirty organizations that included representatives from healthcare, nursing, physician groups, medical device manufacturers, and public health and consumer advocates. The goal of the briefing was to gain more bill sponsors. By its conclusion, every member of the Caucus had signed on.

My second trip back to DC lasted two days with a more challenging goal. The Senate bill, identical to the House version, took longer to gain support, especially from Senate Republicans. Knowing bipartisan support would be needed for passage of the bill, I set out to meet with the staff of key Republican leaders to raise awareness around the need for sharps safety reform and to enlist the support of more bill sponsors. Over two days, I met with senior staff of eleven key Republicans, including Rep. Cass Ballenger (R-NC), who would later prove to be essential in advancing the bill.

Republican leaders and their staff in the Senate repeatedly raised similar areas of concern as they considered the bill. Their concerns included: the additional financial burden imposed by new regulations on hospitals within their constituency, particularly those situated in rural areas; employer resistance based on a perceived lack of cost effectiveness; and resistance to any legislation that isolated them from other Republican colleagues in the Senate. Most expressed these concerns even before being offered any background of the bill.

Strategies that seemed to reduce resistance a bit included sharing my story along with evidence demonstrating that safety device adoption reduced injuries and follow-up costs. In addition, it was important to share that individual pricing for devices was expected to go down as utilization became more commonplace with widespread industry adoption.

Regulatory and Legislative Victories

In October, Senate bill cosponsors Senators Reid (D-Nevada), Boxer (D-CA), T. Kennedy (D-MA) and Jeffords (D-VT) helped lead floor debate. Within a month in November of 1999, two key victories occurred. For the first time, OSHA introduced an updated BPS compliance directive recognizing safety sharps as the primary line of defense against SIs, driven by compelling evidence that injury rates had been reduced across 300 hospitals using safety sharps. Violations of the new directive would result in fines being issued by OSHA compliance officers. Second, a new alert titled: "Preventing Needlestick Injuries in Healthcare Settings" (NIOSH 1999), which focused attention on the requirement that employers needed to involve frontline workers in SI prevention efforts was published by the National Institute of Occupational Safety and Health.

Although both actions represented progress, there was little assurance that employers would comply with the new directive for several reasons. First, employee complaints, which most typically triggered on-site enforcement visits by OSHA, were rare. Next, no fiscal resources for the enforcement of the new directive were provided to OSHA. Based on its current budget, that meant OSHA could afford to make a single unannounced hospital visit once every seventy-five years. Lastly, it could take as long as ten years to implement an updated BPS through non-statutory channels. Over that time, it would not be unreasonable to anticipate many more hundreds of thousands of workers could experience preventable SIs.

By May of 2000, Democratic Senate and House sponsors for HR 1899 had grown significantly. Unfortunately, the same was not true of sponsors on the Republican side. The Congressional logjam did not mirror what was happening in states around the country, where visibility and legislative support for action had grown considerably. Since 1998, when California first passed legislation, ten more states had enacted laws designed to reduce SIs. Twenty other states introduced legislation during that same period, including my home state of Massachusetts, which became the eighteenth state to enact SI prevention legislation. Given the critical mass of state activity related to SI prevention across the country, it should have signaled to Congress the need to enact federal reforms to better protect workers. Regardless, it appeared to have little effect on the Republican leadership in Congress.

Throughout this time, ANA worked persistently with the media to keep the issue of SI prevention on the front burner. One day, an ANA Government Relations staff member received an unexpected call from the chief of staff for Rep. Ballenger. She informed the ANA staff member that her sister, who was a nurse, had sustained what she believed was a preventable needlestick injury at work. She was aware of ANA's advocacy on the issue and, in the event she could convince Rep. Ballenger to hold a hearing, asked whether ANA would be willing to provide testimony at the hearing. Of course, ANA agreed.

About a month later, on June 22, a Congressional hearing was convened before the bipartisan Committee on Workforce Protections, a subcommittee of the Committee on Education and the Workforce. The hearing was convened to hear testimony on whether the recently issued OSHA compliance directive was adequate for improving injury protection for healthcare workers. I was asked by ANA to provide testimony on its behalf. Aside from my testimony for ANA, others invited to speak before the congressional committee included the chairman of the Frontline Healthcare Workers Safety Foundation, the Assistant Secretary of OSHA, a senior HIV and infectious disease consultant from Kaiser Permanente, a representative of the Service Employees International Union, and an epidemiologist from Wayne State University.

The congressional hearing room was crowded and included members of print and television media. Those of us offering testimony were seated together at a table facing members of the committee. After introductions and opening statements from the chairman, Rep. Ballenger, and the ranking minority co-chair Senator (Sen.) Owens (D-NY), testimony began. In my testimony, I shared my personal story and argued on behalf of ANA that the current BPS compliance directive was inadequate, and that congressional action was necessary in order to better protect healthcare workers from injuries like mine.

The witness testimony and subsequent questions from committee members covered a wide range of issues, including asking why, if the compliance directive contained provisions that mirrored the bills currently before Congress, was the bill necessary? Another focus of questioning by the committee was the extent to which the directive protected US healthcare workers. Testimony made clear that OSHA directives did not cover public sector workers. In addition, despite demonstrated efficacy, safety sharps devices were still only in use within a small percentage of US hospitals. Finally, the limitations of current funding levels for OSHA enforcement of the compliance directive were discussed, allowing for inspections to be conducted in about two percent of US hospitals annually.

By the end of the hours-long hearing, both Rep. Ballenger and Sen. Owens expressed a new understanding of the serious potential health risks associated with preventable SIs. In addition, rather than rely simply on the rollout of the BPS compliance directive, they both agreed there was a need to utilize statutory reforms to better protect at-risk workers in a timelier fashion.

What followed over the next few weeks was remarkable. Rep. Ballenger, who was now championing our legislation, assembled key stakeholders, including the ANA, AHA, device manufacturers, healthcare worker unions, and other cosponsors. Together, they met and agreed on language for a new bill entitled the Needlestick Safety and Prevention Act. On October 4, I watched on C-Span as Rep. Ballenger spoke at the microphone to move the bill's adoption by the House, and in the absence of any dissenting voice, the bill passed by unanimous consent.

Just twenty-two days later, on October 26, I was leaving MGH after one of my appointments with Eric when the MNA beeper I carried went off. I called the office, and the executive director's executive assistant informed me that Senator Kennedy had called and left a phone number requesting that I call him back. I dialed the number she gave me, and a person answered saying, "Senate floor." For a moment, thinking I had transposed the numbers, I almost hung up. Instead, I told him I was trying to reach Sen. Kennedy.

He said, "Sure. He's right here." A moment later, I heard Sen. Kennedy's voice: "Karen, the Senate just passed the bill by unanimous consent, and I wanted you to be the first to know. It's on its way to President Clinton's desk."

The Needlestick Safety and Prevention Act Becomes Law

As exciting as that news was, ANA staff understood the value of a public signing. Throughout this eighteen-month campaign, they had taken advantage of every opportunity to raise public awareness around the need for reforms to prevent SIs. This occasion would be no different. Thirteen days later, on November 6, 2000, I was present in the Oval Office alongside sixteen other stakeholder group leaders to see President Clinton sign the bill into law. It was a special moment—one I will never forget.

As the culmination of what felt to me like many years of advocacy, the bill had become law relatively quickly after being filed in Congress. Many things came together to make the new law a reality, not the least of which was a critical mass of support across the country from nurses, stakeholders, an engaged media, and ANA leadership. In my mind, the enactment of these new worker protections would not have happened without ANA. And I would not have had the opportunity to add my voice and face to the issue of SI prevention without my involvement with my state nurses association or ANA.

As he signed the NSPA into law on November 6, 2000, President Clinton made the following statement:

> ... *The Needlestick Safety Act makes clearer the responsibility of employers to lessen the risk of injuries to workers from contaminated sharps devices. It also encourages manufacturers of medical sharps to increase the number of safety devices on the market. This legislation will help make health care occupations safer.*
>
> —**The American Presidency Project 2000**

President Clinton's statement placed proper emphasis on some of the important reforms that would need to take place going forward, both within the medical device marketplace and healthcare arena, in order for sharps safety to be enhanced in the future for healthcare workers.

Leadership Reflections

When I became a nurse in 1973, I envisioned a career that would be spent entirely in direct patient care. It was the place I felt the most satisfaction as a nurse and where I thought I could make the greatest impact on patients' lives. At no time could I ever have imagined having to confront the life or career-altering consequences I faced as the result of my workplace injury. When I think about how close I came to not reporting my injury when it occurred, I feel a tremendous amount of gratitude. It is entirely plausible to think that a failure to report my injury could have resulted in a serious delay in diagnosis and initiation of treatment for two potentially lethal bloodborne infections. I certainly could never have personally afforded to assume responsibility for the financial burden associated with my care.

Leadership is defined in many ways. One of my favorite definitions—and very relevant to my leadership in this arena—comes from research conducted by the Center for Creative Leadership. The Center defines leadership as "a social process that enables individuals to work together to achieve results that they could never achieve alone" (McCauley 2024, 1). I carry with me a perpetual sense of gratitude that I had the professional and personal support systems in place at the time of my injury that allowed me to venture beyond my individual circumstances and put a public face to the issue of SI prevention.

To that end, I will always feel grateful to family and friends who played a part in my journey as well as my professional association, the American Nurses Association, which made it possible for my voice and story to be amplified around the country and enabled me to join with other nurses and healthcare workers to help bring about needed reforms for SI prevention. It remains my personal belief that passage of the NSPA and revisions to the BPS in 2001, as well as related safety reforms in Massachusetts, would not have occurred without ANA's leadership and involvement.

Given the persistent gaps and progress yet to be realized in the arena of SI prevention, my personal passion related to worker safety continues to the present time. I feel it every time I have a conversation about workplace safety. I feel it as I engage with others who continue their commitment to reducing SIs by promoting systematic injury surveillance and data analysis that allows us to monitor progress and reduce gaps. And I cannot help but feel pride in the tangible progress I see every time I have my blood drawn and witness a worker made safer by having access to a safer sharps device designed to protect them from injury.

As a nurse leader who had a hand in helping make the workplace safer for others, I feel grateful for those opportunities. My greatest wish is to see nurses and other healthcare workers take advantage of the many tools that have been put in place through policy change to keep them as safe as possible. It remains my firm belief that when workers are safe, patients are safer—and that, in order to optimize patient safety, the healthcare industry must do everything possible to prioritize worker safety.

Chapter

8
▼

Forging a New Career Path

The flurry of activities I found myself engaged in during those early years following passage of the new federal law included travel to speak before healthcare providers and administrators, as well as providing testimony before numerous state legislatures related to SI prevention. Between 2000 and 2002, I was invited to speak to various audiences in more than sixteen US states and six countries outside the US. It wasn't long though before I found myself feeling restless and looking for a different path to pursue in my nursing career.

As someone accustomed to maintaining some control over my life and career, the restlessness and the uncertainty I felt about my future was not an easy space for me. That was despite the fact that I was doing well relative to my HIV and HCV treatment. Repeated negative testing indicated I could consider myself cured of HCV and that my HIV was undetectable on a stable and well-tolerated medication regimen. Still, I knew I would not be returning to direct patient care. I had not handled a sharp in the years since my injury and could no longer envision myself doing so. I knew I needed to find another path back to nursing where I could utilize my skills, knowledge, and experience.

Internal Unrest at the Massachusetts Nurses Association

I remained active in my state nurses association, but it was not the Massachusetts Nurses Association (MNA) I had led as president since 1997. Internal tensions between close to twenty thousand labor members and the rest of the membership divided the association over whether to continue our affiliation with ANA.

Labor members were nurses represented by an MNA collective bargaining unit within their employment settings. All were covered by contracts that defined terms and conditions of employment negotiated by collective bargaining representatives and ratified by their members. MNA membership also included nurses who were not organized under a collective bargaining agreement.

Labor members viewed ANA as too moderate and slow to respond to nursing's critical concerns. MNA members loyal to ANA insisted that state affiliation was essential for representing the interests and needs of nurses in Massachusetts. They viewed ANA as a representative voice for nurses in all roles and at all educational levels, as well as a strong and respected national proponent for the promotion of safe patient care, safe practice environments, and ongoing educational advancement.

The foundation for internal dissension and unrest exhibited by MNA labor members had been laid over several years. It culminated in a contentious and difficult membership fight. After the initial defeat of a disaffiliation vote taken by thousands of members at the World Trade Center in the Boston Seaport district, labor members of the MNA succeeded in their efforts to disaffiliate from the ANA in March of 2001. Despite the labor membership's claims that MNA disaffiliation was motivated by ineffective advocacy by ANA, from my personal perspective, the movement was a power and resource grab. Their actions destroyed a respected and longstanding ANA-affiliated state professional association with the sole intention of forming a national union.

Months before the actual disaffiliation took place, disenfranchised MNA leaders who remained loyal to ANA began laying the foundation for a new 501(c)(3) nonprofit, driven by the belief that labor members would eventually accomplish their goals. Marie Snyder, a nurse attorney and longtime MNA member loyal to ANA, led the charge to help us define the new organizational structure and bylaws and meet other necessary legal requirements. Papers were filed with the state and IRS the day after the second disaffiliation vote to incorporate a new ANA state-affiliate that was soon approved by the ANA board.

I served as the first president of the new ANA state association in Massachusetts to provide members with some continuity in the face of much anger, sadness, and disruption. I felt all those emotions too, but while the professional commitment I continued to make as a state nurse leader represented an important and ongoing obligation in my life, it did not fulfill my own need to find a new way forward for myself.

Educational Advancement

My pursuit of education beyond my basic diploma program at Catherine Labouré shaped my career perspective. It had taken me ten years to go back to school to pursue an undergraduate nursing degree. I was one of those diploma grads who long resisted the idea that additional education would make me a better nurse. It was a clear lesson in not knowing what you don't know. I had no ability at the time to understand that advancing my education would not simply broaden my perspectives on life but also change the nurse I was and could become.

My initial return to school for my Bachelor of Science in Nursing (BSN) arose from pressure I felt in my workplace. Expectations were growing within my hospital and clinical setting that BSN education was a necessary pursuit for nurses in direct care. After long consideration of my options, and after speaking to a nursing faculty member I knew from my diploma program who now taught at Curry College, I chose to enroll in Curry, which was located near where I was living at the time. For a number of reasons, that choice turned out to be a pivotal one.

Over the next two years, I attended classes while continuing to work weekends in the ED. At about the same time as I began my BSN program, an attending physician at the Brigham named Tom Lee, with whom I had worked throughout his time as a medical resident, contacted me. He and another Brigham attending physician were conducting a chest pain study at the Brigham and recruited me to be one of their research nurses. Although I had never been a research nurse before, I accepted the job knowing my role would involve working with Tom, along with helping to enroll and follow up patients presenting to the ED with chest pain.

I met requirements for completion of my BSN in 1985, taking advantage of classes along the way that offered leadership content. Very unexpectedly, at graduation I received the Nursing Award given for peer leadership and consistent academic and clinical excellence. Also unexpectedly, it was in my BSN program where I was introduced to a nurse faculty member named Mary Manning who would soon become a career-long mentor and dear friend.

Following my graduation from Curry, I returned to my practice in the ED and continued for another year as a research nurse on the chest pain study. As a member of the research team, I would attend meetings every other week to discuss study progress, patient enrollment, and ongoing data analysis. While simultaneously serving as a Brigham attending physician and the study co-investigator, Tom was also pursuing his Master of Science in Epidemiology at the Harvard School of Public Health (HSPH). Listening to his discussion of epidemiological principles related to the chest pain study methodology and data analysis at our meetings, Tom inspired my interest in pursuing a graduate degree in public health. Following completion of the study in 1986, I enrolled in the MPH program at Boston University. Tom has remained a good colleague and friend to this day.

It was not long after I began my MPH program that I started to appreciate how foundationally complementary the values and principles of public health were to the practice and basic tenets of the nursing profession. I completed my MPH within two years. Along the way, I took advantage of other opportunities to work as a research nurse—first on an infant mortality study being conducted at the HSPH, and following graduation as the project coordinator for a trauma registry project also conducted at the HSPH. In the early 2000s, I also served as a project principal on the Nurses Education Hepatitis C Project at the MDPH and concurrently as an HCV Advisory Committee member for the MDPH.

In 2002, after being advised by Mary that "it was time for me to return to school," I enrolled in the dual degree graduate program in Boston College Connell School of Nursing to pursue my Master of Science in Nursing (MSN) and PhD. My original thinking was that, upon completion of my MSN, I would teach nursing in a university setting while completing requirements for my PhD. In the end, I never sought a teaching position as other career opportunities took me in a different direction.

After going back and forth between the dual curricula for three years, including spending time at the MDPH to meet the necessary clinical hours requirement for my MSN and meeting my obligations as a doctoral research fellow, I began work on my dissertation. My doctoral dissertation focused on the lived experience of nurses who sustained SIs—an area based on my review of the literature that had never previously been studied. I successfully defended my dissertation in March of 2010 and, at the school commencement ceremony, was surprised to receive the Connell Commencement Award.

Mentorship and Leadership—No Success Without Others

By the time I completed my PhD requirements at Boston College, I had been a member of the ANA board of directors for close to two years. Circumstances leading to my election to the ANA board in 2008 are memorable for me and set me on another unexpected career path. I share this story often, particularly as I speak to younger nurses or whenever I am teaching undergraduate classes or content on leadership.

I received a call one day from another Massachusetts nurse leader named Barbara Blakeney who was a past president of ANA. She and another past ANA president, as well as the current ANA president, had created a tradition of spending time together every year over President's Day weekend.

Barbara said to me, "Karen, I have good news and bad news for you. Which do you want first?" Asking for the good news first, she responded: "Becky, Ginna, and I think you should run for a seat on the ANA board."

I said, "What's the bad news?"

Barbara said, "Your nomination papers are due in two weeks."

I completed and submitted the required paperwork in time, campaigned, and was elected to the board seat at the next ANA House of Delegates. To this day, I consider myself fortunate to count Barbara, Becky Patton, and Ginna Betts among my most valued mentors and friends.

Mentorship is often and rightfully linked to the process of leadership development. Over the course of my nursing career, I have felt fortunate to be the direct recipient of support, advice, and insight from more experienced nurse mentors. They have supported my career in countless ways, including helping me see myself in ways I never could have envisioned, inspiring me to pursue opportunities I might have allowed to pass by, and helping me to realize my full potential as a nurse leader.

Based on my experience, I believe no success is realized alone or by accident. It is mindful and intentional activity—the result of hard work, careful listening and presence, constant learning, perseverance, and passion for what you are doing or choose to do. Seeking out mentors along the way is a necessary part of becoming an effective leader.

Additional Professional and Leadership Advancement: 2002-2010

I have felt so fortunate and blessed throughout my career. While I can comfortably acknowledge and feel personal pride in my accomplishments and the contributions I've made over many years, I have also been fortunate enough to receive public recognition. Some of that recognition represented milestones that helped advance my leadership career prior to my election as ANA president in 2010, including the award of a doctoral fellowship at the Connell School of Nursing. That fellowship helped defray much of my tuition expense and made pursuit of a PhD possible.

My induction as a Fellow into the American Academy of Nursing in 2006 expanded my network of nurse colleagues and leaders whose work and accomplishments continue to inspire me. My recognition as a Living Legend by my state nurses association as well as a distinguished alumna at Boston University's School of Public Health were also meaningful acknowledgments of my leadership.

While there are nurse leaders who prefer private over public recognition or honors—I have had my own moments when I fell into that category—public recognition can serve as an important source of inspiration. Part of what leaders do is to inspire and ignite passion and purpose in others. I hope I have been able to do that in some small measure for other nurses throughout my career.

Leadership Reflections

My career experiences have admittedly been broad. I do not want any nurse who is reading my story and envisioning a future as a leader to compare my path or the nature of my career with your own. You will determine your own path and future. As I share my career details, I think it is also important that I share how I was able to take advantage of opportunities I pursued such as educational advancement and voluntary board positions.

It never hurt that I was single and had no other major time or family commitments that coincided with assuming new leadership opportunities in my life. That is not to say a nurse needs to be single to explore or take advantage of such opportunities. Certainly, I have seen and worked with many nurse leaders who accomplished much while they also had family and other personal commitments. In those cases, support from a partner, spouse, or significant other becomes important and necessary.

It is also important to understand that whenever you assume leadership roles on either a voluntary or paid basis, your time commitments can be significant. As you would plan for any expansion of your life responsibilities, it is important to understand what is involved, along with any associated costs or expected income. Until I was elected ANA president, most of my leadership commitments including board service were voluntary.

Academic education is also a costly endeavor, so you need to understand what options exist for helping to defray costs and other associated expenses. Most of all, make sure you feel passionate and motivated relative to the choices you make.

Chapter

9
▼

ANA Presidency: Part One

People often ask me what being ANA president was like. My response has always been the same: it was the hardest and the best job I've ever had. Despite my many years as an active nurse leader in the ANA state affiliate, it was not until I joined the ANA board in 2008 that I was truly able to begin to appreciate the talent and dedication of ANA staff.

The breadth and depth of expertise and passion they brought to their work on behalf of members and the nursing profession spanned a wide range of issues impacting nurses in practice. ANA advocacy encompasses workplace health and safety, leadership, scope and standards of practice, code of ethics, workforce development, and social and public policy, among others. Through that critical work and collective power, ANA represented the interests of more than 2.6 million employed registered nurses in 2010. Becoming ANA president gave me an even clearer sense of its importance and potential.

Election as ANA President

My path to being elected president of ANA in 2010 was the result of another series of events that I never could have predicted. You would think by this time I would have become accustomed to things happening unexpectedly in my life. While that wasn't necessarily always the case, I had by then learned to be open to new life experiences.

The circumstances surrounding my election began with a call I received one evening in December of 2009 from a group of ANA leaders with whom I served on the board. The purpose of their call caught me totally off guard—encouraging me to run for ANA president.

As I listened to those members on the phone, so many thoughts were going through my head. I had barely completed my first term as a director on the ANA board and had never considered service beyond that. There were also sitting board members who had served for longer periods and who seemed to me to have the experience and desire to run in the upcoming election. In addition, I was still working on writing my doctoral dissertation. But rather than immediately dismiss the idea out of hand, I listened to what they had to say and why they felt so strongly.

At the end of the conversation, and aware that the election would be held in June at our House of Delegates (HOD), I responded by saying, "If I am able to complete and defend my dissertation by the end of March, I will run." Encouragement from other members was the only thing that could ever have led me to seek the ANA presidency. However, my immediate priority had to be finishing my dissertation.

I successfully defended my dissertation within that self-imposed deadline. Not long after, I began taking steps necessary to launch my campaign for ANA president including completing nomination papers, putting together a campaign committee, soliciting my campaign manager, selecting a fundraising chair, and developing messaging for my campaign. In June of 2010, as a current board member, I traveled to Washington DC to attend the HOD. Members of my campaign committee, along with my younger sister Ruth, traveled there to provide on-site support for my campaign.

The final ballot included five candidates for president—unusual for an ANA presidential election. Three of the candidates on the ballot, including myself, were current board members. The other two were a former board member and a former state association executive director. Given the constituencies of support for each individual candidate, there was a potential for the election outcome to create divisions within the ANA membership beyond the election outcome. Each individual candidate had secured support from members of their own state or region.

Aware that any candidate's election could split the membership, the five of us came together and created a statement of unity that each of us signed and then presented to the House delegates prior to any voting taking place. The statement included a public commitment that, regardless of the election outcome, the prevailing candidate would have the unconditional support of the other four. It was an important step for us to take to ensure a smooth transition for the newly elected leader as well as for the association moving forward. To me, it modeled the epitome of leadership and unity for our members.

Most on-site campaigning for all ANA elected positions took place within a large, designated space in the hotel. Candidates for office or their campaign representatives would typically meet there with voting delegates at designated times over several days; there were also candidate forums and regional state delegate meetings where invited presidential candidates could respond to questions and share a future vision for the association. Voting took place the morning of the day before the HOD adjourned.

After being informed the night before that I had been elected, I was announced as the newly elected 35th president of ANA at the final session of the House the following day. It was customary at the HOD for the incoming ANA president to briefly address the members before adjournment. While I had campaigned for the office and learned of the election results the evening before, nothing had prepared me for that moment. ANA had a long and proud history of advocating for its members and the advancement of the profession. ANA presidents before me, all of whom I respected and admired, had served selflessly and with distinction and vision on behalf of the profession. As I stepped to the lower dais to address the HOD, I could not help but feel the weight of the responsibility I would be assuming.

There is a picture of me being sworn in that easily takes me back to that moment looking like a deer caught in the headlights. I can still remember feeling anxious, proud, and excited all at the same time. I also recall my flight back to Boston the next day and thinking about how my life was about to drastically change.

It is a humbling experience to become the leader of such an important nursing organization because you know this isn't just about you. What's tied up in an election like that, especially at the highest level of an organization, are the hopes and needs of members and the profession itself. I came to appreciate that fact even more deeply over my time as ANA president. The good news was, as alone as I felt in that moment, I would not be alone in my efforts going forward over my subsequent two terms as the elected leader of ANA.

As the HOD concluded, I joined the board and ANA CEO Marla Weston in another room to call my first board meeting to order as president. That was followed later in the evening by a meeting with the ANA General Counsel to make board-level service appointments for various committees such as the ANA-PAC. Then the real work began—starting with two landmark events that set the tone and agenda early in my presidency.

Passage of the Affordable Care Act

The backdrop against which I began my presidency was historic. In recognition of ANA's significant contributions to the passage of the Affordable Care Act (ACA) under the leadership of my predecessor, Dr. Becky Patton, President Obama had made an appearance at the 2010 ANA HOD. My work served as a continuation of what Becky and other past presidents had accomplished related to healthcare reform, culminating with the passage of the ACA, which was guided by a vision referred to as the "triple aim" for better access, better care, and lower cost for patients.

Every ANA president, to some extent, carries forward work from previous presidents. An old adage originally attributed to Isaac Newton in 1675 states, "If I have seen further, it is by standing on the shoulder of Giants" (letter correspondence to Robert Hooke, 1675). Nothing could be truer with respect to leaders who have served as ANA president. Something that each of us came to learn once elected was that making positive progress, especially relative to health policy reform, is a time-consuming and iterative process. The most important thing is to keep moving forward.

As I traveled around the country to speak to members about the ACA and what it meant for nurses as well as patients, I also reminded them of ANA's decades-long efforts to advocate for high-quality, affordable healthcare as articulated since the early 1990s in *Nursing's Agenda for Healthcare Reform* (ANA 1991). In partnership with dozens of other nursing organizations, ANA had long been focused on a broader healthcare agenda that encompassed strong support for preventive care and universal access for all Americans.

True to that commitment and counted among ANA's proudest moments in its long history, was its leadership as the first and only healthcare organization to step forward and endorse the Social Security Amendments of 1965—the legislation that established the Medicare and Medicaid programs. And beyond the triple aim of the ACA, *Nursing's Agenda for Healthcare Reform* encompassed a fourth aim—to ensure an adequate supply of a skilled workforce to promote consumer access to a range of competent providers, including registered nurses.

It makes sense, therefore, that one of my first priorities during my first two years as ANA president was to educate members about the benefits of the ACA for their practice, patient care, and healthcare access. I frequently discussed the ACA and highlighted its provisions in numerous presentations to ANA members. The new law not only enhanced patient access to healthcare but also enabled nurses to more effectively advocate for patients' rights and needs. In addition, it mirrored core healthcare reform principles widely promoted by ANA since the 1990s.

Launch of the Institute of Medicine Future of Nursing Report

In November of 2010, just a few months into my presidency, the landmark Future of Nursing report was released by the Institute of Medicine (IOM), offering a way forward for addressing some of the changes proposed in the ACA. Titled *The Future of Nursing: Leading*

Change, Advancing Health (IOM 2010), the report reflected two years of evidence-based work that captured the value proposition for healthcare attached to ensuring that the scope of the role of registered and advanced practice nurses encompassed the full extent of their education and training. Together, passage of the ACA and launch of the FON report largely set the agenda for much of my leadership and outreach efforts, particularly during the first two years of my presidency.

Internal Governance: ANA Board of Directors

The ANA president serves as the association's chief elected officer. In contrast to other board positions, and commensurate with the overarching responsibilities and full-time nature of the role expectations, the ANA presidency is a paid position. Nurse leaders who typically seek the position are longtime members of ANA. Many have served as state presidents as well as members of the board and understand the nature of ANA's long and impactful advocacy on behalf of members and the nursing profession. Those who run to serve as ANA president do so in order to champion the issues that matter most to nurses and promote safe, quality patient care.

Two of the inherent and immediate responsibilities of every ANA president as the elected leader and primary spokesperson of the association is to lead its governance as chair of the board of directors and to facilitate annual meetings with the ANA House of Delegates. A critically important part of leading the board is to build a sense of community and shared purpose. My predecessor, Dr. Becky Patton, spoke often about the stages of successful coalescing of board members. The first stage, *forming*, was the process of bringing members of the board together, which, in the case of ANA, is determined by the outcome of the election at the House of Delegates.

During this initial stage, part of my responsibility as president was to assure new board members were provided with the support, resources, and information necessary to orient them to the organizational structure as well as board role expectations and responsibilities. Based on Tuckman's model, additional stages of maturing the groups' development included: *storming, norming, performing,* and *adjourning* (Tuckman and Jensen 1977, 419).

As important to me as anything else in this multistage process was socialization of board members. One of my favorite aspects of this work was to identify a group social activity together with members of the ANA executive team each time the board met in Washington DC. Some of the activities I helped plan included trips to downtown DC to visit historic memorials, the White House, or a Washington Nationals baseball game. We even spent one evening at a glow-in-the-dark bowling alley in downtown Bethesda, Maryland that turned out to be one of my favorite nights out with board and staff. As a leader building a team, I believe fun is important too.

Early in both of my terms, I leaned heavily on the CEO and the General Counsel to help ensure the successful onboarding of those newly elected members who joined the board. I was mindful that a shifting board composition related to staggered terms could also shift the group dynamic and effectiveness. Newly elected board members can bring a varying range of leadership and governance experiences as well as skill sets to their position.

As president, it was necessary for me to assess those strengths and gaps and to work to ensure that the needs of new board members were met on an individual and group basis. In some cases, I helped mentor individuals to promote leadership growth and group synergy. In other cases, I worked with the CEO to identify staff resources that would be needed along the way to develop a strong team mentality and sense of shared purpose.

To optimize my effectiveness as president, I understood how critically important it would be for me to develop a close working relationship with the ANA CEO who, as ANA's chief staff officer, works for the board and was responsible for all ANA operations. From the outset of my presidency, I devoted time and energy to developing and nurturing that relationship. At the time of my election, Dr. Marla Weston had been in her CEO role for only a short time. One of the first things I did to make sure we were on the same page relative to expectations tied to our respective roles was to draft a document similar to a memorandum of understanding that set clear expectations between us regarding things like open, honest, and transparent communications. I also took advantage of Marla's knowledge of ANA's operational and strategic initiatives to identify resources that would help me become better informed in my role. Over time, our relationship evolved and grew stronger, contributing greatly to my effectiveness as ANA president.

ANA Constituent State Associations

One of the most critical measures of my effectiveness as the elected leader of ANA was my relationship with constituent member associations where nurses from every state and US territory were represented. Based on ANA's modified federated structural model in 2010, the state associations were the members and individual nurses constituted the state association membership. Therefore, travel to the state associations and meeting with their nurse leaders and members became paramount to my role.

In addition to regularly scheduled calls with state presidents, communications with members occurred during those visits as well as through columns I wrote for the ANA journal and newsletter. As ANA president from 2010-2014, I did my best to listen to and amplify members' concerns and to act on them through board action or policy initiatives using ANA's resources at the national level.

Another opportunity for the board to hear from members and identify important trends impacting nursing occurred at a two-day annual gathering of state association presidents and executive directors at the Constituent Assembly (CA). ANA would host the meeting, but the agenda was set by an elected executive committee of ANA state leaders and was facilitated by the CA chair.

While CA meetings provided a clear opportunity to identify common ground across constituent associations, it was also an opportunity for divergent trends, issues, and concerns to be raised by the assembly. Often they related to differences in geo-political influences. Despite that, CA represented an important opportunity to chip away at and come together around painfully divisive issues like collective bargaining. During my presidency, I witnessed how that dynamic contributed to greater understanding and unity among members.

Another invaluable partnership for me as president was the opportunity to connect with elected and staff leaders of more than thirty-five national specialty nursing organizations through our organizational affiliates (OAs) program. Marla and I met annually with our OAs at an all-day meeting hosted by ANA that I facilitated prior to the annual HOD. Our meeting discussions offered invaluable insights into issues of significant importance to the broader nursing community and resulted in a number of joint partnerships and initiatives. During my presidency, I had the opportunity to speak to many nurses who were members of specialty organizations and helped expand the number of our OA partners.

ANA HOD and ANA Reorganization

In 2010, ANA's highest governance structure was our annual HOD, a meeting over which I presided as president that was attended by over 625 elected constituent state delegates. Organizing each HOD meeting involved countless moving parts and significant ANA operational resources. Planning for the next meeting by ANA staff commenced with the adjournment of the present HOD and represented a significant association financial commitment every year, including travel subsidies for delegates.

Among the predominant challenges and responsibilities of elected association leaders serving on a board of directors is an obligation not only to meet fiduciary obligations, but also to create a strategic vision that assures relevance, responsiveness to member needs, and future sustainability of the organization. In the summer of 2011 at my home on Cape Cod, my main beach reading was a recently published book focused on building greater efficiencies and relevance within membership associations.

That book was titled: *Race for Relevance: 5 Radical Changes for Associations* by Coerver and Byers (2011). The authors examined strategic and operational challenges faced by associations and offered advice on how greater success might be achieved. Recommendations were focused on creating a radical cultural transformation that would enable greater association relevance and sustainability. Among them were eliminating redundancies, building simplified organizational structures and processes, and strengthening the value proposition for members.

I returned to ANA headquarters in September inspired by the possibilities put forward in *Race for Relevance* (RFR) and wanting it to be read by all association leaders. I began by bringing a copy to CEO Marla Weston, who read it and then disseminated copies of the book to all her staff as required reading. I did the same with the ANA board. In February of 2012, Marla and I led a day of strategic planning by the ANA Board with an eye towards initiating a major transformation across the association. In advance of our strategic planning, ANA staff provided the Board of Directors members with a draft proposal based on recommendations from RFR.

Once buy-in among ANA board and staff were apparent, our work shifted to bringing our constituent state associations on board. As president, I spearheaded that critical work with in-person travel to the states and frequent webinars, messaging, and calls with elected state leaders that allowed time for questions and discussion. Despite some lingering resistance shared by some state leaders about initiating such rapid change, the end result was a complex web of bylaw changes reflecting a more streamlined and effective governance structure being brought forward to the 2012 HOD. By initiating the most substantive changes to ANA in more than three decades, we hoped to transform the association into an organization that was more relevant, responsive, and sustainable for our members.

The first morning of the 2012 HOD bylaws session was a heavy lift for me as the presiding officer. Association leaders, including those at CA, worked together to tweak proposed bylaw amendments that were multi-tiered and interrelated and would require consideration at a special session of the House. To move forward with proposed changes, delegates would need to approve more than seventy pages of bylaws that would upend our current governance structure within a predetermined two-hour time frame. For anyone familiar with Robert's Rules, it was a huge undertaking.

In the end, the majority of proposed changes to our structure were adopted. I was proud that the entire association came together and demonstrated its willingness to take what I believed were necessary risks to promote the growth, relevance, and sustainability of the ANA.

Reflections on Internal ANA Leadership Activities

Organizational governance is not the most compelling or sexy reading content. But the investment of time and energy in good governance over both my terms represented some of the most important leadership activities in which I engaged as ANA president. Good governance and respectful, open communications laid an important foundation not just for a more direction-focused organization, but also for building members' trust that the association and its leadership were acting in their best interests.

One of my first internal leadership activities as president involved taking steps to assure that board members operated with a clear sense of shared understanding, responsibility, and purpose. In addition to assuring resources were provided to accomplish that end, it was important that I modeled behaviors I wanted to see from my board members. I can recall one board meeting in the middle of my first term when it became evident to me that, despite being provided with in-depth background reading in advance to help spur readiness for discussion on an important agenda item, a particular board member once again came unprepared to the meeting.

As she interrupted the board discussion to ask for a recounting of background on the issue, I could feel myself silently losing my cool. Knowing it was important not to do that, I turned to my first vice president and asked her to take over facilitation of the meeting discussion while I stepped out of the room to regain my composure.

Leaving a board meeting while in session was not something I had ever done before, but it was the right thing to do. After the meeting was adjourned, I sat with that board member to share my concerns about her lack of preparation. As I recall, it never happened again. It was one example of numerous opportunities I had to work with board members during my presidency and help guide their leadership development.

It can be challenging to lead a large membership organization, particularly one where geographic and political realities divide the membership. As I traveled around the country to speak to and meet with members, it was also my experience that members often brought specific expectations to our one-on-one conversations. Perhaps the greatest lesson for me as president under those circumstances was to listen carefully and respectfully to what members were saying or asking for and bring that info back to the board and CEO as feedback without making any judgments, promises, or commitments in the moment. Sometimes, that is not as easy as it sounds.

My final reflection on my internal ANA leadership activities relates to the radical governance transformation that took place during my presidency. Prior to ever reading *Race for Relevance* on that Cape Cod beach, I can remember having numerous conversations with the CEO about association relevance and sustainability. At the time, ANA—not unlike other membership associations—was struggling to evolve and grow. Our association had not kept pace with realities of the larger healthcare environment. Our value propositions, especially for younger generations of nurses, were not attracting many new members and our current workflow processes could be time-consuming, labor-intensive, and financially burdensome. However, it wasn't until I read the book that a light bulb went off and I began to clearly see new possibilities for growing our membership and building greater association efficiencies and relevance for practicing nurses.

Having said that, it was remarkable that we were able to garner so much support for such radical governance and structural change across a large membership association over an eight-month period. To accomplish that, carefully designed communications and open member engagement were key. We used all the communication and digital media tools at our disposal—email, webinars, websites, print and e-newsletters, face-to-face meetings, and conference calls. We were also responsive to question and answer online postings as well as areas of most concern to our state associations.

There were important leadership lessons learned throughout the entire process. There was a need to lean in as a leader who was committed to the needed change, along with an understanding that, in such a large and diverse organization, governing could not occur by consensus. Regardless, the need to listen and balance the needs of all stakeholders was paramount.

Perhaps the most important lesson for me as an association leader was not being satisfied with the status quo and being open to taking calculated risks and embracing change for the future good. The next chapter relates to my leadership activities as ANA president with external groups and partners.

Chapter

10

▼

ANA Presidency: Part Two

I have found it challenging to find a way to offer a glimpse into external leadership activities during my four years as ANA president without creating an intolerably long chapter. Rather than try to summarize major events that occurred, I am including a description of some of the activities I engaged in that I believe contributed to my ability to lead ANA effectively.

Beyond my governance responsibilities, as ANA president I served as the official representative and chief spokesperson of the association. My position would take me from US states to the White House and include meetings with healthcare, business, and policy leaders around the country. I also traveled to countries around the world to meet with international leaders. There were many opportunities for me to interact with public media and health policy leaders, including some within the Obama administration.

The first order of business as I began my service as ANA president was to take advantage of the many tools and resources afforded me to prepare and grow as an ANA leader.

Early Preparation for My New Role and Responsibilities

I began by reviewing recommended background reading to better familiarize myself with current ANA initiatives and the organizations with whom I would be engaging in my new role. I was quickly overwhelmed by hundreds of unfamiliar organizational and healthcare acronyms, among them: AAHSA, AAPCC, AHRQ, AOA, APC, ASPE, BPC, CDR, CMG, CMMI, ASTP, and ECRI, to name a few. My need for a glossary quickly became evident.

As I read through background materials, I also created a list of topics, priorities, and external relationships that would require more in-depth reading and staff briefings to bring me up to speed. Requests for staff support went through the ANA CEO, since there were clear boundaries from the outset of my service between operational staff and strategic volunteer leadership. Based on my prior leadership experiences, I was fortunate to have a pretty clear understanding of those boundaries. I was also fortunate that ANA employed some top nurse experts I could access with questions about a broad range of issues relevant to my needs.

Media training was another important aspect of my preparation. ANA had an outstanding public relations and communications team who oversaw my training. One of the things I had to quickly overcome in my new role was my dislike for having my picture taken. I have often joked in the years since my time at ANA that I had learned to default to an "ANA smile" whenever being photographed. In particular, I disliked having professional make-up done before going on camera as I never felt like my authentic self. I am also not sure I ever grew to enjoy doing media interviews, but I realized it was an important part of my role as the chief spokesperson for the association.

To further my role preparation, I also set up formal and informal meetings with Marla Weston, the ANA CEO. Marla and I would meet in her office as well as outside of ANA headquarters on an informal basis to discuss numerous issues. Early in my presidency, she also accompanied me to provide support as I traveled to outside meetings and scheduled events. I also created and utilized an informal group of advisors. Individual advisors were selected based on the different strengths and insights they could bring. I also trusted that each would maintain strict confidentiality as I considered difficult issues or critical decisions.

Individuals I chose included past ANA presidents, select members of my board, and people outside of the organization whom I trusted to offer honest feedback and input. In the end, there were many decisions that I would need to make alone on behalf of the association, so having support and hearing a diversity of opinions was important to my decision-making process. For many organizational leaders, the nature of their role and responsibilities can leave them feeling isolated and lonely at times. I was one of them.

As time progressed, and as a jam-packed daily calendar became the norm for me, it would soon be necessary to have my executive assistant block time every week for additional reading as well as reflection. I recognized pretty quickly after my election that both were becoming a luxury for me, but would be necessary for me to function at my best in my role.

It was time well-spent to better prepare myself as ANA president. Taking walking breaks a couple of times a day between meetings and calls to get some exercise and clear my head didn't hurt either.

Personal Advocacy and Leadership Priorities

Beyond advancing established ANA strategic priorities, as ANA president I was afforded many opportunities to connect with nurses around the country and engage with them about issues they identified as being important. Opportunities also existed for incoming ANA presidents to set and pursue priorities of their own. I was reminded during an interview I did a few years ago that, unique to my background and based on my almost twenty-six years of caring directly for patients prior to my election, I had the longest period of experience as a direct care nurse provider of any ANA president.

I believe those years of direct care experience provided me with a deep understanding and unique insights into the daily challenges faced by nurses. Beyond that, my injury experience created a profound appreciation for the hazardous nature of nurses' work and elevated nurses' safety to the forefront of my own leadership and advocacy work—particularly preventable occupational injury and illness. From my perspective, workplace safety for nurses and other healthcare workers is about much more than SI prevention. It is my firm belief that safe working environments are essential for the delivery of safe, quality patient care. It also requires more attention by employers not only to workers' physical safety, but also to their mental health.

Among the health and safety issues I prioritized during my presidency were workplace violence and safety, nurse bullying and burnout, preventable injuries related to patient movement and handling, inadequate nurse staffing, and exposure to hazardous drugs. Making progress relative to each issue required a thoughtful, multi-tiered strategy responsive to existing conditions within the healthcare and socio-political environments. In some cases, strategies might include: raising awareness on an issue with policy leaders; initiating a summit to promote brainstorming; updating professional practice or ethical standards; making visits to Capitol Hill to advocate for new legislation; or offering testimony to advance existing legislation before Congress.

It had also long been my belief that, in spite of nursing's long history of advocacy for healthcare reform, not enough had been done to optimize the scope of practice for registered nurses (RNs). One ramification of that was a chronic underutilization and undervaluing of the competencies and abilities of RNs who provide direct patient care within the healthcare system. While one of the key messages within the IOM's Future of Nursing report explicitly stated that all nurses should practice to the full extent of their education, knowledge, and scope, compelling supporting evidence dictated that the report's first recommendation be focused specifically on advanced practice registered nurses (APRNs).

Evidence of the impact of RN care on patient safety, quality, and outcomes did exist at the time, but additional efforts were needed. Identifying new care delivery models could accelerate opportunities for demonstrating, capturing, and amplifying the larger policy conversation around the impact and value of RN care. Patient care transition and care coordination were among the well-defined but underutilized healthcare roles suited to the competencies of experienced RNs.

Two aspects of that important work during my presidency related to efforts to advance educational reform and baccalaureate entry to practice for registered nurses. This involved participation in discussions with other nursing and policy leaders to influence and promote a shared vision for needed change related to RN education. It was during this period that efforts were made to facilitate RN matriculation from associate degree to BSN programs.

Another key effort was ANA's participation in the Coalition for Patient Rights, a group focused on preserving APRN scope of practice. The group represented over thirty entities and was formed to counter extensive efforts by the American Medical Association (AMA) to promote misinformation about the meaning of the full scope of APRN practice. The Coalition's activities also countered AMA's attempts with state legislators around the country to limit the practice scope of APRNs.

Nurses' self-care was another important focus and priority for me as president. I was always struck as I attended or spoke at large meetings by the visual impression that so many nurses appeared to be overweight. Based on that anecdotal evidence, however, I could not determine if it was representative of the entire profession. One of the opportunities I took advantage of as ANA president was to meet periodically with co-investigators of the *Harvard Nurses' Study* (HNS) in an advisory capacity.

The HNS was one of the largest and most impactful longitudinal study of women's health in the United States since it was established in 1976. During one of the meetings I attended with study co-investigators, it occurred to me that a snapshot in time of the nurses' health data might serve the nursing profession. At my request, study co-investigators agreed to release that summary data to ANA.

The results confirmed suspicions that many of us had relative to the overall state of nurses' health in this country—at least at this one point in time. We weighed more, exercised less, smoked more, reported greater levels of stress, and ate less nutritious diets than the average woman during this same time in the United States. Follow-up nurse surveys conducted by ANA staff over the next several years confirmed trends brought to light by the HNS data.

In more recent years, survey results from more than 24,000 nurse respondents indicated, against the backdrop of COVID, threats to nurses' mental health had also increased significantly (Cuccia et al. 2022, 352). Inspired by results from the HNS data and its survey findings, ANA launched a new programmatic initiative in 2017 called *Healthy Nurse, Healthy Nation*™ designed to engage nurses and provide resources to help improve personal wellness. ANA outreach to nurses and employers around the country and provision of free resources to help improve nurses' lifestyle and mental health and promote healthy behaviors resulted in participation of more than 340,000 nurses and 600 organizational partners during the first five years of the program.

Federal Healthcare Policy Advocacy

Those familiar with my policy journey after my SI in 1998 might assume that my policy work began there. In actuality, it began much earlier and was tied to my engagement with my state nurses association. As I described in an earlier chapter, I joined my professional organization right out of my nursing program and became an active member in the mid-1970s at local and state levels. It was my involvement early in my professional career that began my appreciation of the value proposition of membership in my professional association.

Later, as a state association leader, I developed relationships with my state legislators and would personally advocate as well as offer testimony at hearings focused on issues impacting nurses in Massachusetts. I participated in activities like the annual Legislative Days at the State House, meeting state legislators face-to-face, and offering public testimony. Those experiences all helped prepare me for policy work later on a broader scale.

ANA's standing as a well-respected professional organization that offered healthcare expertise as well as critical policy leadership created numerous opportunities for me to interact with leaders on the Hill as well as within the Obama Administration. Within a week of my election, I found myself at the White House as an invited guest to a ceremonial event hosted by Vice President Biden to showcase and celebrate the reauthorization of his landmark legislation, titled the Violence Against Women Act (VAWA). In addition to enhancing services for victims of sexual assault, domestic violence, and stalking, VAWA provided funding for expanding victim advocate, criminal justice, and judicial services. Each of those initiatives is closely aligned with ANA's priorities related to holistic women's rights and healthcare.

I would characterize my healthcare policy work as ANA president at the federal level in several ways that include: representing ANA at ceremonial White House events such as the one I just described; offering Congressional committee testimony in support of initiatives such as expanding Title IX funding for nursing education, as well as advocacy for growing the number of nurse-managed clinics which provided access to healthcare for vulnerable populations; and face-to-face meetings with members of Congress as well as Obama Administration-appointed officials and staff.

Early in my presidency, I scheduled in-person meetings with several key members of the Obama Administration including the Centers for Medicare and Medicaid Services Administrator, the Deputy Secretary of Health and Human Services (HHS), and the Director of the Agency for Healthcare Research and Quality. Each of these meetings allowed me not only to introduce myself, but sometimes offered an opportunity to raise and discuss issues of importance to nursing and ANA. With that in mind, I met with ANA staff to discuss priorities relevant to the office prior to each scheduled meeting.

Occasionally, unexpected things happened as a result of those efforts. One example was a personal invitation I received for a follow-up meeting with President Obama's chief of staff. Another meeting I attended, along with other healthcare leaders, at the invitation of Vice President Biden followed the horrific Sandy Hook Elementary School shooting in 2012 to discuss gun control through a public health lens. Sadly, I was the only nurse in attendance at that meeting—something that was still too often the case and needed to change if nursing was going to be successful in amplifying its voice and growing its policy influence.

As ANA president, I was also included in more happy and celebratory events as a guest of the White House for the annual Christmas parties as well as for President Obama's inauguration upon the occasion of his reelection—both coveted invites.

Fostering Open Communication, Collaboration, and Working Partnerships

ANA engaged in numerous partnerships and collaborations during my presidency with many involving outside nursing and healthcare organizations. As president, one group on which I represented ANA was the Tri-Council for Nursing which at the time, aside from ANA, was made up of the elected and staff leaders from leading national nursing organizations including the American Association of Colleges of Nursing (AACN), the National League for Nursing (NLN), and the American Organization of Nurse Executives (AONE—now AONL). Focusing beyond the priority concerns of any single organizational member, Tri-Council meetings were convened with the goal of building consensus around issues impacting the entire nursing and healthcare community.

Consensus building efforts would often result in joint statements being issued by Tri-Council members. It was also not unusual after a particular deliberation for organizational collaborations to result. Two examples of Tri-Council collaborations during my presidency took place between ANA and the National Council of State Boards of Nursing (NCSBN) as well as one that emerged at the urging of the Robert Wood Johnson Foundation (RWJF). Neither of those organizations were members of the Tri-Council at the time, but each would periodically be invited to attend meetings to inform the membership around particular issues.

The collaboration between ANA and NCSBN emerged relative to a recurring issue with recent grads as well as staff RNs posting inappropriately on social media about patients or their employers. RNs who posted inappropriately were often surprised when disciplined by their employer or their state board of nursing. What did not exist for nurses at the time were clear guideposts around professional standards of behavior relative to the use of social media. On behalf of ANA, I worked with the NCSBN executive director to help create and disseminate explicit guidelines for RNs using social media.

The second collaboration example related to an opportunity presented by RWJF, who offered to convene several meetings between leaders of national nursing organizations represented on the Tri-Council, as well as two nurse practitioners from the NP Roundtable and leaders of five national physician groups. On behalf of their medical organizations, those physician leaders had expressed opposition in writing to the first recommendation put forward in the IOM's Future of Nursing report advocating for removal of barriers to enable the full scope of practice for APRNs. I represented ANA in those meetings.

Over a period of several months, the organizational leaders agreed to engage in a facilitator-guided dialogue related to interdisciplinary collaboration and to discuss specific concerns raised by physician group leaders. Conversations were frank and difficult at times, but always respectful. Ultimately, all leaders reached agreement on several areas that were captured in a final draft document titled *Common Ground: An Agreement Between Nurse and Physician Leaders on Inter-professional Collaboration for the Future of Patient Care*.

Nurse and physician leaders were then asked to take the draft joint statement back to their respective organizations for broader board approval in late 2011. The final outcome was incredibly disappointing, though, as all nursing organization boards approved signing onto the statement while all physician group boards refused to support it. With that outcome, hopes that the joint statement could serve as a launching pad for both healthcare disciplines to move forward together in a more collaborative fashion were dashed.

International Advocacy

My international advocacy most typically occurred during meetings convened by the International Council of Nurses (ICN). A federated structure, the ICN is composed of national nurses associations from more than 130 countries. Rather than advocating on behalf of nurses within our respective countries, actions taken at ICN meetings focused on advancing nursing's global impact and reducing barriers to nurses' full scope and safe, quality practice worldwide.

As the international member of the ICN representing the United States, I traveled to numerous countries around the world on behalf of ANA to meet with other national nursing association leaders. Between 2010 and 2014, I attended ICN meetings in Canada, Sweden, Ireland, Japan, Malta, and Australia. My experiences at ICN were incredibly eye-opening, providing unique opportunities to meet with nurse leaders around the world to discuss global healthcare delivery as well as the scope and issues surrounding nursing practice within and outside of the United States.

My appointment from 2011 to 2014 as a nursing representative of a non-government organization [ANA] acting in an advisory capacity to the US delegation at the World Health Assembly (WHA) provided another unique international leadership experience. Held annually in Geneva, Switzerland, the WHA is the deliberative and decision-making body of the World Health Organization comprised of about 194 member countries across six world regions. The US delegation is typically chaired by the Secretary of Health and Human Services, who during my years was Secretary Kathleen Sebelius.

Among the health topics advanced in WHA deliberations and resolutions in my years as a delegation member related to: a vision and strategy for global immunization; smallpox eradication and destruction of variola virus stocks; mechanisms for control and prevention of cholera, polio, and malaria; strategies for safe water management; climate change and health; strengthening the healthcare workforce; improvement of health through safe and environmentally sound waste management; neglected tropical diseases; pandemic influenza management; and consideration of the social determinants of health relative to promotion of global health.

Reflections on External ANA Leadership Activities

Effective leadership can be demonstrated in many ways. Good leaders exhibit similar qualities with respect to how they openly communicate, influence, inspire, advocate, build trust, problem solve, and engage with and treat others. The work I was so privileged to be a part of in my role at ANA was incredibly challenging but also rewarding. Along the way, I learned new leadership lessons that reinforced my approach to leadership while at ANA. I plan to share them in the next chapter.

I believe solutions for improving healthcare won't come simply in the form of new technologies or medications. Rather, they will be based on things like promotion of positive and safe, healthy work environments and the effectiveness and valuing of nurses' contributions, regardless of role or setting as they practice to the full extent of their license.

Additional solutions lie in actions taken to improve patient experiences. Those include efforts taken to enhance the meaningful nature of healthcare encounters, efforts to support patients' participation in their own healthcare, and coordination of health services in places where people live, work, and play. I hope my work and leadership at ANA contributed in some small part to making progress in some of these areas.

I know all leaders want to leave a legacy behind. For me, it is less about what I accomplished, but rather how I might be remembered as a leader. In retrospect, I carry with me so many memories of those years and that work. I was honored during my presidency to receive prestigious public recognition for my health policy advocacy efforts, as I was counted among *Modern Healthcare's* "Top 100 People in Healthcare" as well as the "Top 25 Women in Healthcare." Subsequent to my service as ANA president, I was also gratified to be awarded two honorary doctorates. I have no doubt that both reflected, at least in part, on my time and leadership at ANA.

Perhaps one of my most lasting memories as a leader happened after I adjourned my last Membership Assembly (previously House of Delegates) as president and was waiting for a taxi in the hotel lobby to take me to the airport. My executive assistant found me in the lobby and approached me to say, "President Daley, I just wanted you to know that you were the kindest person I ever worked for." To this day, that moment remains one of my most special memories.

Chapter

11
▼

Leadership Lessons Learned

As you read this book, I hope to help you understand that leadership is as important during direct patient encounters as it is in the C-Suite. Nurses in leadership positions have the ability to garner critical resources and set strategic priorities related to care and practice. Nurse leaders providing direct care can make a huge difference not only in the patient experience, but also in the quality and outcome of the care received. Nurses who lead in partnership with patients and their families are also well-positioned to influence the environment in which care occurs.

Today's nurses are being challenged in so many ways. Healthcare workflows and processes of care that impede safe, quality patient care can be difficult to overcome. We need nurse leaders and the insights they bring from direct engagement with patients and other caregivers to promote needed change.

Choosing to build a career focused on achieving a leadership position requires the pursuit of advanced education as well as a broad range of experiences that equip you with the necessary depth and breadth of skills and knowledge. My advice is to take some time to discover what you want to accomplish for yourself. Let your passions be part of what guides your choices, and seek out experiences that align with your career goals.

For nurses exploring their path to leadership, there is no one-size-fits-all all. Consider ways you can advance your knowledge, education, and experience. If you decide to go back to school to pursue further education, explore options that represent the best fit for you with respect to your passions, schedule, and program affordability. Do not allow tuition costs to deter you. There are available subsidies in the form of scholarships, fellowships, and loans. My tuition for graduate school at Boston College was largely defrayed by a fellowship award. Otherwise, I could not have afforded to pursue doctoral education.

In addition to advancing your education, seek out volunteer or paid leadership opportunities to pursue. Join and get involved with your professional as well as your specialty nursing organization to allow you to grow and network. Volunteer for committees within your practice setting. Connect with nurses you view as professional role models. Identify and establish a relationship with potential mentors who are willing to support and guide your future growth.

My legacy of leadership emerged from several things: the intertwining of my lived experiences, observations, and continuous learning; exposure to the mentorship, role modeling, and ways of being of other more experienced nurse leaders; and taking advantage of opportunities that were opened to me, sometimes at the generous urging of others. All of these influences helped me grow and mature in my critical thinking, leadership skills, and development as a nurse.

Throughout previous chapters, I have shared memories and moments from my personal leadership journey. This chapter will focus on lessons I have learned that have guided me throughout my career. The initial leadership lessons are related to my involvement in public policy change, including actions taken within the legislative arena. Those are followed by lessons learned or reinforced during my time as ANA president. I conclude with some general lessons that represent learnings spanning my entire career.

Don't Underestimate the Power of Your Voice

Always remember that your voice matters and that a collective voice is stronger than a solitary one. Collectively, our voices represent political influence. Throughout my career, I have experienced the benefit derived from speaking up as an individual as well as from joining others in advocating for a common good or goal. Build teams or coalitions to move your vision forward. Finally, always remember that facts, evidence, and personal experiences all matter. Personal stories are especially powerful.

It's Not Enough to File a Bill

Passing legislation can take time—anywhere from months to years. Efforts to create change through legislation take patience, planning, and vigilance. Strategies for success include identification and education of key legislators on both sides of an issue and mobilizing a broad base of support. In my efforts to garner support for the federal SI prevention bill, I met with legislators who both supported and opposed the bill. However, even with passage of a bill, it doesn't ensure the intended change occurs. Unfunded legislative mandates as well as lack of enforcement both impede the intended impact of newly enacted laws. Resources are needed for implementation, oversight, and enforcement of laws. It is also important to realize that not every problem warrants a legislative approach.

Your Experience and Practice Make You an Expert on Nursing Practice and Healthcare

Since 1990, with the sole exception of 2001, nursing has been ranked in annual Gallup polls as the most ethical and trustworthy profession. Nurses are also viewed as credible sources of information and guidance on health policy issues. Regardless of the experience or position of a particular state legislator or member of Congress, most can benefit from education on issues impacting nurses, patients, and healthcare. Establishing personal relationships as a constituent of your lawmaker enhances your access and ability to inform them.

Politics is Not Simply About Lawmakers Passing Legislation

Politics are about governing, public policy, and the allocation and control of resources. Sometimes filing legislation is appropriate to the public need. At the same time, while bills may be filed to create new laws, they can also be filed to give voice and prominence to an issue and to sway, inform, and build support over time from lawmakers. I have seen many examples of this approach in action, especially at the level of state politics.

In some states like Massachusetts, ballot referendums represent a means for enabling citizens to bypass the state legislature by collecting enough signatures to place legislative initiatives on the voting ballot. Even unsuccessful ballot referendums can generate a significant amount of public debate and visibility around an issue that may sway public opinion over time.

Timing and Synergy Around an Issue can be Important in Politics and Public Policy

The lack of evident or voiced support for changing public policy or passing legislation translates into likely failure. Without indications that constituents, stakeholder groups, or other legislative leaders support passage of a bill, there is little hope that it will be released for consideration beyond the initial public hearing or committee. Timing and synergy matter for many issues.

At the time bills on SI prevention were under consideration by Congress, many stakeholders and constituents as well as the media had brought support and visibility to the issue that was impacting healthcare workers around the country. Personal stories like mine were key to progress made in adding Democratic cosponsors to the bill. However, it was hearing testimony offered to a powerful Congressional committee that broke through the divide and created a tipping point that generated bipartisan support for subsequent passage by unanimous consent in both the House and Senate.

Be Willing to Take Calculated Risks for the Good of the Organization

The lessons that follow emerged for me during my time as a state and national association president. As ANA president, I was no longer acting simply as an individual nurse, but as the elected leader of a national organization. That role shift changed the lens through which I viewed and acted on behalf of nurses, patient care, and ANA. Many of these lessons relate to my experiences during the transformation of ANA. That transformation process involved proposing major structural changes to increase the efficiency and effectiveness of an organization whose members prided themselves on its long traditions and history. Prior to my presidency, the last changes to ANA structure had taken place in 1989 during the pre-digital age.

When elected leaders, including myself, put their support behind radical changes to the ANA structure and the way it did business, there was significant resistance voiced by the membership. It was a risky endeavor. We faced a range of membership responses—from skepticism to doubt to anger and support. Much of the resistance stemmed from the rapid timeline proposed for mobilizing around and adopting structural changes through bylaw amendments at our 2012 House of Delegates.

Among the things at stake were the trust and support of the members and my re-election as ANA president. We spent several months engaging in a multi-pronged effort presenting our strategic vision to members, correcting misinformation, gathering feedback, and finally moving forward to the House with over seventy pages of bylaw changes. What drove our efforts, however, was the realization that making these changes represented the right direction for our organization. Our central message was that we were striving for the good of the whole, not just the national organization.

To Encourage Change, Repeated, Consistent, and Multi-Channel Communication is Imperative

This lesson was front and center as part of our process of being as transparent as possible as we presented the proposed framework and strategic vision for ANA transformation to our board and membership. A carefully designed communication and member engagement plan was key to our success. It was not possible for us to over-communicate about the radical changes we were proposing.

Over a period of four months, we utilized every communication tool at our disposal to reach members including regular conference calls with state elected and staff leaders, print and e-newsletters, online messaging boards with Q&A postings, leadership webinars, pairing of ANA staff and board members with state association leaders, and on-site visits to speak directly with state members. Careful listening and attempts to be responsive to members' concerns about proposed structural changes were critical. All the time and effort invested paid off as most recommended changes to the ANA governance structure were adopted at our June House of Delegates.

Don't Ignore the Squeaky Wheels or Assume Silence Means Agreement

It was important to get objective feedback from all stakeholders as we engaged around implementing dramatic changes that would impact the whole of our organization. That meant, particularly on our calls with state leaders, soliciting feedback from everyone. In some cases, we learned we had more support than expected. There were also opportunities to directly hear and respond to expressed concerns. Most of all, we learned never to assume silence meant agreement.

Change Frequently Originates at the Grassroots Level and May Not Follow a Specific Plan

In the end, nurse leaders from within the membership worked together before the House of Delegates convened to create and bring forward alternative bylaw proposals that addressed lingering concerns. Those compromises allowed most proposed changes to occur and made the association transformation a reality.

I will conclude my list of leadership lessons with more general but no less critically important things I have learned during my life and career.

Authenticity as a Leader is Key

Being honest and open as a leader and keeping commitments you make by doing what you say you will do are important qualities. They establish trust and credibility in you as a leader. When I embarked on the work to transform ANA, I benefited from the trust and goodwill the membership and other leaders were willing to extend to me based on our histories and past dealings with me as a leader.

It is Difficult to Feel Gratitude and Anger at the Same Time

I can largely attribute learning this lesson as I sat and listened to others share their experiences in Al-Anon meetings years before my needle-stick injury occurred. Earlier in this book, I shared details about my family background growing up in a dysfunctional home with two alcoholic parents. Despite my relatively high functioning abilities in my professional life, in my thirties, I became aware of persistent resentment and lingering anger towards my parents—especially my mother. Although I was uncertain at the time where it came from, I knew I had some unfinished business to deal with relative to my parents.

To gain needed insight, support, and begin healing, I sought out individual psychotherapy. It was in those sessions that the suggestion was made that I attend Al-Anon to gain clearer understanding of how I was affected by my parents' alcoholism. Soon I began to understand the ways I had been affected by my parents' drinking and behaviors. It was in those meetings that I also came to appreciate how important it was to live with gratitude rather than resentment and anger.

Over time, it became second nature for me to start my day focusing on appreciation for all the good things and people in my life. Even after my injury, I was able to focus on how fortunate I was rather than allowing myself to be overwhelmed with feelings of anger or feeling sorry for myself.

Emotional Intelligence is an Important Quality for Leaders

Emotional intelligence is a key competency that we know makes clinical nurses more effective in their role. The same is true for great leaders. My ability to sense and understand the emotions of those around me no doubt began developing in my childhood as a means for self-preservation. Beyond my childhood, though, it served me well in my care of patients and in my interactions with other leaders. The good news is that emotional intelligence is a competency that can be developed or learned at any point in your career.

Always Focus on What is Right for Patients and Care About Other Nurses

Regardless of where I have been in my career, I have always felt grounded in my own beginnings and experiences as a clinical nurse. My priorities were related to what is most important for patients as well as those who provide care. That became an especially important north star as I led ANA. While the issues ANA faced and advocated for were varied, my focus was always on doing what was right for patients and nurses.

Take Time for Reflection

Developing self-awareness with respect to your own needs is a critical process that promotes personal and professional growth. Self-awareness serves not only as a means for helping you identify your own career paths and goals, but also for better understanding your strengths and the areas that need growth.

Our lives are busy, and it's easy to get caught up rushing from one thing to another. Making time for yourself on a regular basis, away from the busyness, to allow time for quiet consideration of your needs as a person and leader is paramount. It did not take long after I was elected ANA president for me to realize that every minute of my day was being scheduled away. My decisions as an ANA leader became more well-thought-out once I set aside regular time to take walks and time for reflection. It is also a key strategy for overcoming adversity.

Seek Out Leadership Opportunities

Don't wait for leadership opportunities to come to you. Seek them out for yourself. It took me some time to learn this lesson. Good places to start in your career are volunteer opportunities for joining committees in your employment setting or within your professional organization. Focus on areas of work that you feel passionate about.

Don't Discount What Others May See in You

It is easy to simply dismiss out of hand positive things others might say about or see in you. In the early years of my career, I had an especially self-effacing nature. As I matured, I learned not to be so quick to discount compliments or positive reinforcement from others. Instead, I learned to take in what was being said, particularly by those individuals I respected and who knew me well.

Never Be Satisfied with the Status Quo

My final lesson is an especially important one. Nurses are well-positioned to challenge many aspects of healthcare that need improvement or reform. That includes how our profession practices. So many of the norms in our practice have been rooted in tradition with little thought given as to why we provide care in a particular way. Countless examples of that have existed over many decades. In my own leadership stories, I shared times when it was important to question the processes and structures long accepted as the status quo.

Beyond disruption of current processes, nurses bring the experience and understanding to contribute to the development of new technologies, protocols, and enhancement of approaches to safe care. Beyond processes of care, it is paramount that we ensure that the scope of practice for nurses is guided by demonstration of safety and quality patient outcomes rather than acceptance of restrictions imposed upon us by other professions or policymakers. Only then, I believe, will nursing be able to reach its full potential as a healthcare discipline.

Chapter 12

▼

Conclusion

As is the case for most people, I have faced numerous adversities in my life. It is not realistic to live not expecting challenges to occur. It is the undeniable nature of life. Anticipating challenges and adversity as inevitable provides us all with an opportunity to proactively develop the means to adapt and overcome them. Such anticipation can also help us maintain a more positive and resilient attitude throughout our lives regardless of circumstances we face.

There are things that can help ease the burden of navigating life's adversities. Having a social network and support system is huge. Being open to asking for help and keeping in perspective that difficult times will eventually pass also makes them easier to get through. I wish I could say I was always wise and experienced enough, particularly in my younger years, to take advantage of some of this advice. But life is about learning, and sometimes failure can be our greatest teacher.

A common saying that I first heard in Al-Anon meetings is: *Insanity is doing the same thing over and over and expecting different results.* While I might not have ever reached the insanity threshold, I was often guilty of using the same approach over and over to deal with emotional difficulties and adversity in my life.

In my early nursing career, I compartmentalized struggles in my personal life while continuing to experience growth as a nurse clinician and leader. I have no doubt, however, that the feelings and difficulties I experienced on a personal level seeped into my professional life. I simply had less awareness that it was happening at the time. Similar to my ability to compartmentalize the risk posed by my SI from my ongoing health struggles, I was still able to perform well professionally. That fact was reinforced by public recognition I received starting at my nursing school graduation and continuing throughout my professional career.

I have been privileged with the many opportunities I have had to grow as a nurse leader. I also feel blessed that I have had opportunities that allowed me to experience and grow from personal adversity as part of the process of overcoming them in my personal life. And while I did not always appreciate the difficult nature of the challenges I faced at the time, overcoming each of them made me a stronger and more resilient person and leader. They also led me to embrace a different kind of humility, understanding, and healing.

Personal Adversities and Overcoming Them: Surviving My Childhood

I believe we all do whatever is necessary as children to survive. In my case, that meant protecting myself from the emotional hurts and neglect I felt. I learned not to trust my parents to be responsive in an appropriately emotional or nurturing way. As a result, I became a child that needed little. I became self-reliant and independent in the face of not being able to depend on my parents for what I needed. Acting like I needed no one and nothing from my parents became my way of getting through those years even though I wanted their love and validation.

Not unlike children of divorced parents, in my failure to make the situation better I felt a sense of responsibility and blame for my parents' dysfunction. As pervasive fear and the stress of uncertainty dominated my home life, I created a resilient self that allowed me to survive. Once I moved on to living my own life, I thought I was leaving that dysfunction behind. Without realizing it, though, the same traits I developed that allowed me to survive a difficult childhood emerged later as part of my own adult dysfunction. They also created the need for a second overcoming in my life.

Emotional Struggles in my Mid-Thirties

Successes I realized early in my adult life as a nursing student and practicing nurse only served to mask what I would eventually recognize as problematic. My independence, self-reliance, and the sense of responsibility I demonstrated were considered positive attributes in a nurse. On the other hand, the emotional dysfunction that was becoming apparent in my personal relationships, including around my parents, took time for me to recognize as a problem.

Talking with my brother Kevin about what I was feeling was the first step in helping me validate my experiences as a child. When I finally reached the point of being willing to ask for help, it came in the form of therapy and Al-Anon. It was in therapy that I began to experience my real feelings for the first time. Once I let down my guard, there weren't many sessions in which I did not cry. The hurt was deep. Journaling and expressing my emotions out loud also became important tools for processing them. Much of my anger, resentment, and emotional distancing covered my hurt and sadness. As I described my own behaviors and the sense of responsibility I carried and acted upon as a child, I realized I'd never had a real childhood. I needed to acknowledge all the ways I had been affected before I could begin to work on making changes.

The process of healing from my childhood wounds has been a long and gradual one for me, and I don't always get things perfect. I can revert at times to old mindsets, behaviors, and patterns, but I am much more likely to recognize and acknowledge them when they happen. My personal self-awareness and willingness to live my life differently represent my second emotional overcoming. I am no longer simply surviving to live, but doing my best to allow myself to trust, love, and depend on others.

My Workplace Injury

When my injury occurred, I was in a wonderful place caring for patients. Emergency departments can be chaotic and pressure-driven environments. At that point in my career, I believe I was experienced and confident enough to provide care that was safe and high-quality for most patients I cared for in the ED. I had also reached the point where providing direct care and support to patients and their family members gave me more satisfaction than the adrenaline rush of caring for a patient in the trauma room or someone in cardiac arrest. I still keep a box filled with notes of gratitude written by a patient or their family members. Those meant more to me than any award I've received. Sometimes when I felt particularly tired or discouraged as a nurse, I pulled them out and read them to remind myself why I had chosen nursing.

The day my injury occurred was otherwise quite ordinary. Even after it happened, I was more irritated than alarmed. The nature of the exposure did not seem to me to be high risk. Learning five months later that I had been infected with two serious bloodborne viruses was shocking as well as frightening for me.

I think the uncertainties I felt were the hardest things to deal with. I was uncertain what the impact on my health and life would be. I was uncertain what side effects I would face from the potent drug regimens. And I was uncertain how effective they would be, although my physician, Eric, had reassured me from the beginning that the HIV could be managed over the longer term. The trust I placed in him allayed my fears regarding the physical effects of prescribed therapies, even as I suffered significant side effects.

The psychological impact of being infected with HIV and HCV posed a different challenge for me. The decision I made not to return to patient care was the correct one, but it also left me feeling lost and disconnected. My identity seemed no longer tied to my work as a nurse. Rather, my identity had become my illnesses. My professional identity and my life as a nurse seemed so far away from the day-to-day reality of blood draws, appointments with Eric, and the all-consuming worries about test results.

Several months later—once my health and test results started to stabilize—I shifted my energy and focus to advocacy efforts to legislate needed safety reforms. In retrospect, I recognize those many months of activity served as part of my psychological overcoming of my injury. Not only did it offer me a new purpose and meaning, but it also filled a vacuum of time following my injury. I needed time to adjust to my new reality and to figure out what was next for me in my life.

During that time, I had begun journaling again to process my thoughts and feelings. I also depended on a few people I was close to in my life to help direct me towards a new path as a nurse. Going back to school was a first and key step in that process.

Forging a New Career Path

My final overcoming involved moving beyond my sense of existing in a professional limbo towards finding a new career path into the future. While the safety and advocacy work I was doing were important to me, I knew they did not represent the return to the professional life that I wanted and needed.

Mentors have been important throughout my career. It was one of my mentors, Mary Manning, who listened to my personal struggles and told me it was time to go back to school. By that time, I had earned a graduate degree in public health, but my highest nursing degree was at the undergraduate level. Her advice was the correct advice and I took it. Within months, I enrolled in a dual degree program at the School of Nursing at Boston College that allowed me to pursue a master of science and PhD.

Earning those degrees reinvigorated my career as a nurse. Once again, I felt energized and was positioning myself to explore career options outside of direct patient care. On the ANA board of directors at the time, little did I realize that I was also on the doorstep of finding my next career path as a nurse. As I was finishing up my dissertation research, it was being solicited by other members of the ANA board that spurred me to run for ANA president. The rest is history—literally. Just a few months after defending my dissertation, I was sworn in as the 34th president of ANA.

The process of overcoming has been integral to the person and nurse I have become in my life. My leadership path and career, while a bit unconventional at times, have afforded me countless opportunities to contribute to nursing. I have been extremely fortunate to be the direct beneficiary of wisdom and guidance from many outstanding leaders throughout my nursing career. Nurse leaders have influenced me from the time of my basic education to my years in clinical practice in Boston and beyond.

I don't know what life still holds for me beyond the stories and challenges I have shared here. I do know that behind the scenes were the many people who offered me their wisdom, love, and support. All have allowed me to adapt and move beyond the life adversities I faced.

I will always be grateful to them.

Acknowledgments

An expression often heard today when describing what it takes for children to thrive is "It takes a village." Nothing could also be truer to the process of writing a book. There are so many individuals who helped make the writing of this book possible.

First, my thanks to my publisher Lisa Akoury-Ross and editor Cath Lauria. Both have been incredibly helpful as they educated me in the genre of memoir writing and worked closely with me to capture my personal stories in a way that would bring my feelings as well as experiences to the page. They could not have been better partners. I also want to thank Susan James, nursing professor emerita from Curry College, who edited the earliest version of my manuscript prior to my engagement with Lisa and Cath. Numerous friends and colleagues who shared various career experiences with me took the time to read and provide feedback on specific parts of the book. They include Barbara Blakeney and Mary Manning, as well as Angela Laramie. I also want to thank Martin Greco, a neighbor and fellow writer, who was the first to read through the entire manuscript draft in the midst of the editing process to provide me with his overall impression of the book.

Others served to provide welcome encouragement as my writing progressed. Barbara Goodwyn offered a relaxing space in which to write while I was renting my townhome. Thanks to my sister Ruth Ennis and friends Ellen Burns and Ellen Policow, who patiently listened to me as I provided constant and unsolicited updates on my progress. Also, thanks to Christine Scanlon, who celebrated with me whenever I completed early chapter drafts with dinner at the bar of one of my favorite restaurants on Cape Cod. Finally, thanks to Syd Hale, Karen Pinard, Anne Doyle, and other members of my Cotuit book club for their ongoing encouragement. I look forward to hearing an in-depth discussion of the book at one of our future group gatherings.

About the Author

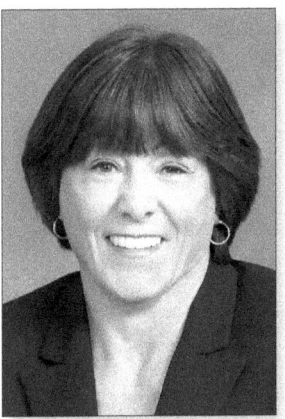

Karen A. Daley served from 2010 to 2014 as the 34th president of the American Nurses Association, the nation's largest nursing organization representing the interests of 3.5 million registered nurses. She has served on numerous boards within her state and national organizations. She is also a current member of the Board of Trustees of the Dana Farber Cancer Institute in Boston, the International Safety Center, and the Barnstable Land Trust. In addition, she holds an appointment as adjunct faculty at Case Western Reserve University.

Daley spent more than twenty-five years in clinical practice at Brigham and Women's Hospital in Boston, including twenty-two years in the emergency department, until she left due to a needlestick injury that resulted in her infection with both HIV and hepatitis C. Since that time, she has been actively engaged on state, national, and international levels in her ongoing campaign to educate others on the importance of sharps injury prevention.

Daley was among those invited to the Oval Office to witness President Clinton sign the "Needlestick Safety and Prevention Act" into law on November 6, 2000.

She has been honored for her excellence in practice and outstanding leadership, and in 2006, was inducted as a Fellow into the American Academy of Nursing. In 2011, Daley was listed among Modern Healthcare's "100 Most Influential People in Health Care" and, in 2013, was selected by Modern Healthcare as one of the "Top 25 Women in Healthcare." In recognition of her global public health advocacy and leadership, she has been awarded two honorary Doctor of Humane Letters.

References

Chapter 5

Johnson, Mahlon, and Joseph Olshan. 1997. *Working on a Miracle.* Bantam.

Chapter 6

Center for Disease Control. 1995. "THE NATIONAL SURVEILLANCE SYSTEM for HEALTHCARE WORKERS (NaSH) Summary Report for Blood and Body Fluid Exposure Data Collected from Participating Healthcare Facilities." *https://www.cdc.gov/nhsn/pdfs/datastat/nash-report-6-2011.pdf*

NIOSH Alert. 1999. "Preventing Needlestick Injuries in Health Care Settings." *https://doi.org/10.26616/nioshpub2000108.*

Chapter 7

Chitturi, Shiuakumar, and Jacob George. 2000. "Predictors of Liver-Related Complications in Patients with Chronic Hepatitis C." *Annals of Medicine* 32 (9): 588–91. *https://doi.org/10.3109/07853890009002028.*

Clinton, William J. 2000. Statement on Signing the Needlestick Safety and Prevention Act. The American Presidency Project. *https://www.presidency.ucsb.edu/documents/statement-signing-the-needlestick-safety-and-prevention-act.*

Holding, Reynolds, and William Carlsen. 1998. "DEADLY NEEDLES/Epidemic's Devastating Toll. San Francisco Chronicle. *https://www.sfgate.com/health/article/deadly-needles-epidemic-s-devastating-toll-2982343.php*

McCauley, Cindy. 2024. "What Is Leadership?" CCL. Center for Creative Leadership. *https://www.ccl.org/articles/leading-effectively-articles/what-is-leadership-a-definition.*

NIOSH Alert. 1999. "Preventing Needlestick Injuries in Health Care Settings." *https://doi.org/10.26616/nioshpub2000108.*

Chapter 9

ANA. 1991. *Nursing's Agenda for Healthcare Reform.* https://www.nursingworld.org/globalassets/practiceandpolicy/health-policy/principles-healthsystemtransformation.pdf.

Coerver, Harrison, and Byers, Mary. 2011. *Race for Relevance: 5 Radical Changes for Associations.* ASAE: The Center for Association Leadership.

Institute Of Medicine. 2010. *The Future of Nursing: Leading Change, Advancing Health.* National Academies Press.

Tuckman, Bruce W. and Mary Ann C. Jensen. 1977. "Stages of Small Group Development Revisited." Group & Organizational Studies 2(4): 419-27. *https://doi.org/10.1177/105960117700200404.*

Chapter 10

Cuccia, Alison F., Cheryl Peterson, Bernadette M. Melnyk, and Katie Boston-Leary. 2022. "Trends in Mental Health Indicators among Nurses Participating in Healthy Nurse, Healthy Nation from 2017 to 2021." *Worldviews on Evidence-Based Nursing* 19(5):352-358. *https://doi.org/10.1111/wvn.12601.*

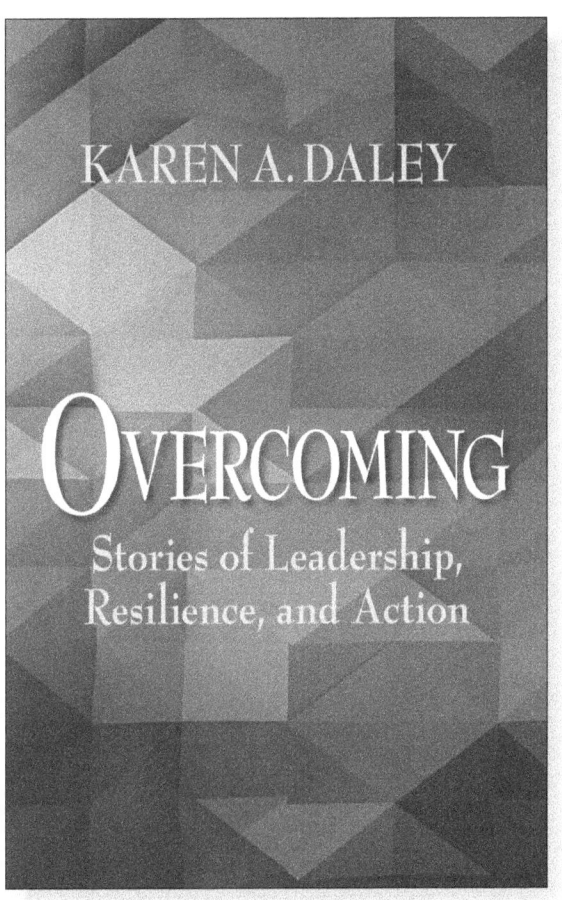

Overcoming
Stories of Leadership, Resilience, and Action
Karen A. Daley
Also available in ebook format

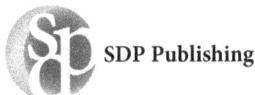
SDP Publishing

www.SDPPublishing.com
Contact us at: info@SDPPublishing.com

www.ingramcontent.com/pod-product-compliance
Lightning Source LLC
Chambersburg PA
CBHW041925090426
42743CB00020B/3448